CRIES
OF THE
SILENT

MY JOURNEY WITH ALS

By Evelyn Bell

ISBN 0-9685383-0-4

1. Bell, Evelyn, 1946- 2. Amotrophic lateral sclerosis--Patients--Biography. I. Amotrophic Lateral Sclerosis Society of Alberta. II. Title.
RC406.A24B44 1999   362.1'9683   C99-910608-2

Photograph on back cover and page 23 by Dean Bicknell, Calgary Herald

Design by Sandra Deren, Excalibur Foxx Ltd.

Printed and bound in Canada

This book is dedicated to my husband,

Larry Bell,

Whose unconditional love and devotion for my care during my illness

Was more than I can ever repay.

I am eternally grateful to him.

Our marriage vows of 31 years ago,
"in sickness and in health" hold steadfast.

You were my strength when I was weak.

You were my voice when I couldn't speak.

I'm everything I am because you loved me.

CONTENTS

ACKNOWLEDGMENTS

First and foremost I praise and thank Almighty God for the strength and courage to write this book and guide my thoughts and words.

My gratitude to my husband, Larry and my mother, Betty for organizing the volunteers so there would be someone here everyday to scribe for me.

My deepest gratitude to my dear friend, Judy Howard for your initiative in acquiring a laptop, scribing and editing this book. Also for your dedication, support and love. Your sense of humor brought sunshine into my life, and your ability to read my mind saved me a lot of energy.

I started the book in August 1998 and completed it in February 1999. This would not have been possible without the help of Bernice Clark, Joan Dauter, Elaine Elick, Shawna Kinniburg, Janie Walton and my niece Janessa Tipton, who scribed this book for me, one letter at a time. I am so very grateful for your support and dedication. I also appreciated your reading to me when I was too weak to point the laser. You were all my partners and you can be proud of your contribution.

Thank you to my sister Sandy Deren for designing the front cover of my book and preparing my manuscript for publication.

Many thanks to Jane Rivest and the ALS Society for publishing this book. It would not have been possible without your support.

I wish to acknowledge, with much love and gratitude, the following people, who have showered me with dedication and love in the past two years. You have helped me look forward to each new day as a gift. You brought joy into my life and love into my heart.

My main caregiver – my husband, Larry – I am eternally grateful for your loving care, especially the many nights that you were at my bedside to make me comfortable. Also for my showers, being my hairdresser and the daily physio you gave me, which made a big difference to my well being. There are so many things to thank you for.

My mother, Betty Schamber for the special foods you so lovingly prepared for me when I was able to eat. Your patience helped me through some rough spots. I appreciate you and all your help when assisting Larry or my caregivers. Thank you for being here to meet our family needs.

Mark Shenfield for bringing the Holy Eucharist every Wednesday morning. Your fervent prayers helped along my spiritual journey. Thank you, Father Bob Kasun and Father John Murphy for saying mass in our home. To Pat Rowlands and Cienne Lenet for their regular prayer visits.

My sister Sandy Deren and sister-in-law Lynda Davidson for your weekly help in putting me to bed, also Lynda's husband Robert for reading to me at bedtime.

The following friends who looked after some personal needs: Kelly Pruden, Elaine Mark, Kim Berry and Samantha Berry.

My sisters Vel Thompson and Laura Barmentloo for the monthly visits that I so looked forward to and for helping wherever it was needed. Peter Barmentloo for running errands. Also thank you Laura for organizing the fundraiser in Lloydminster.

Kon and Brenda Schamber for the massages and meals on wheels.

My brother James Schamber for the ramp you built at the front and sister Joanne Schamber for painting the bedroom.

My friends Adeline and Shannon Leibel and Marguerite Harrison for your regular uplifting visits and help.

Keith and Susan Bell for the special weekend at the Banff Springs Hotel, a very memorable weekend.

Sally and Gerry Stotts for donating your van to ALS for our use. Thank you so much. What a wonderful gift. I am so very grateful for your efforts in spearheading and organizing the Golf Tournament and dinner to raise awareness and funding for ALS, which has now become an annual event.

Mike Klein, Judy Howard, Gary Varti and Joy Gregory for your involvement in the Golf Tournament.

My extended family for your generous Christmas gifts for the past two Christmases.

My nieces and nephews for your unique gift of a star from the Edmonton Space and Science Centre. It really touched my heart.

My uncles, aunts and cousins who donated cash for equipment

and supported the fundraisers.

Doug and Flo Bell, Joan Brown, Marguerite Harrison, and Paul Harrison for your cash donations.

Jane Rivest for your quick response to my questions and needs. I appreciated your emotional support and honesty.

Rachael Owens for the beautiful music which turned my poem into song.

Doctor Labrie for your regular home visits.

My four caregivers: Tina Braun, Bruce Mitchell, Janice Richard and Brian Oishi for your compassion, patience and conscientious care.

Last, but certainly not least, my deepest gratitude to my three sons and daughter-in-law, Derek and Christy Bell, Jarret and Travis Bell for all the times you helped to transfer me, for making me more comfortable in bed or in my chair and for your ongoing encouragement and love.

There are so many people to thank Some were fleeting and some were here to the end.

May God bless you all.

The publication of this book was made possible with the financial assistance of our friends at Medichair Calgary, whose mission is "To provide the best service and products to significantly improve their customers' quality of life".

The committee of the "Tee Off for ALS Awareness" golf tournament are proud sponsors of 'Cries of the Silent'. We are so very proud of you Evelyn!

A TRIBUTE TO MY MOTHER

You were there for me from the start.
You and dad nurtured me to adulthood.
You put love in everything you did for your family;
Your marriage was the role model for your children.

You were there for your grandchildren.
You were there when we needed a break from child rearing.
You were there for me through my two surgeries;
You are here for me now that I have ALS.

Your loyalty and love have no boundaries.
I can't imagine the pain you now feel in your heart,
I can only imagine how I would feel if one of my sons
Had been afflicted with ALS.

You wipe away my tears,
You feed me through my tube,
You assist caregivers when needed.
You do this always with a smile;
I do not hear you complain.

Your patience soothes me through difficult times.
You are there for our family for meals and laundry;
Your baking fills the house with fragrant aromas.
You do this all for love.

I wanted to be the one to take care of you
But God had a different plan.
I love you very much.
I am eternally grateful for all you have done
For our family and me.
I feel blessed to have a mother like you.
Thank you for being with me in my journey.

FOREWARD

"Our theology should enable us to see
God as one in whom we can trust,
even in the middle of the ultimate fear, which is death.
If we laugh in the crisis of death,
that's one way of saying that God is in charge."

Quaker humorist Tom Mullen

My vision of a typical author would be a person hunkered down for countless hours at a word processor, running thoughts through fingertips onto a keyboard. Deleting a sentence and replacing it with a richer thought. Encountering writer's block and abandoning the computer until being further inspired. Writing and re-writing until the manuscript is as close to perfect as it's going to be.

This has not been the case for Evelyn Bell. She hasn't had the privilege of being able to do the simple things that most of us take for granted. Except for the ability to move her head slightly, she is completely paralyzed and unable to speak.

The book you are holding has been written with the use of a laser light, attached to a spectacle frame, laboriously pointing letter by letter to a spellboard and recorded by scribes. Sometimes she was barely able to hold her head up long enough at one time to complete a single sentence.

At times, while scribing, I've seen her head drop onto her chest like a fifty-pound weight. I would cringe and lift her head up and she would carry on. Nothing cooled her desire to write the book that she knew had to be written. A book that would benefit other people with ALS, their families and caregivers. A book that had become her passion.

This book had to be completed while she still had control of her head. There was no time for re-thinking and re-writing. Time was running out. Somehow she was able to put her thoughts together in an extraordinary manner without the benefit of making notes. She stayed organized without the opportunity to read and re-read her text, having to rely on volunteers to read it to her. If she had an inspiration or thought while she wasn't in front of her spellboard, she had to retain it until she was, and somehow she managed to do that.

Evelyn Bell is a perfectionist who always went the extra mile and never took half measures in anything she did. Evelyn would have gone over this book fastidiously if she'd had the ability to do so. Therefore her husband, sons and I wrestled with the idea of having this book edited by a professional. However, when we considered how much effort went into each word in this book, we felt strongly against changing the words that Evelyn had pecked out, letter by letter. This was a labour of love, Evelyn's gift to you. We wanted her thoughts and words, as she was able to communicate them, not someone else's polished prose. We wanted you to experience what she was thinking and feeling in its purest form because this book is from her heart.

It's been an incredible journey and a privilege for me to participate in the writing of this book. The experience has indeed changed me as a person. I looked forward to every moment that Evelyn and I spent together. Walking through her front door, I was always greeted with a smile and the sparkling eyes of a person who had just won the lottery. It is the same for every person who visits Evelyn.

People tend to think that being around a terminally ill person is depressing. It doesn't have to be. Although ALS immobilizes the body, the mind is not affected and those with ALS are still the same people inside as they always were. To spend time with an ALS patient demonstrates living proof that we are not bodies with spirit, but spirits with bodies.

Although the body may have shut down, the essence of the person remains the same. They still cherish the experience of joy and laughter presented to them by the people around them.

Driving to Evelyn's house, I would conjure up thoughts of amusing things that I'd heard or had happened around me or my family so I could share them with her in hopes of making her laugh. It was never a difficult task and she would sometimes go into fits of laughter to the point where her mother would think I was torturing her. Her sense of humour was unalterable and even on those days when she was feeling poorly, we always managed a chuckle or two. Her ability to laugh at herself and find the humour in almost every situation is a memory that will remain with me for life.

Evelyn's undisputed faith in God reveals itself in the manner in which she embraces life in spite of the challenges facing her day after day.

I have learned so much by observing how she continues to live even though she is constantly aware that she is dying. How she sustains her cheerfulness and passion for life is revealed in the pages of this book.

"Cries of the Silent" has indeed been a labour of love. It was written for all of you who are dealing with ALS, as a patient, loved one or caregiver. Evelyn has opened her heart by going inside and revealing how it feels to travel the ALS path. I know it is her hope that the sharing of her experiences and insights will help to ease your journey.

This is her final gift.

Judy Howard

INTRODUCTION

Why am I writing this book?

The most devastating news for those afflicted with ALS is that there is no known cause or cure for this mysterious disease. In addition to this is a lack of public awareness and government funding for ALS research.

Too few people and caregivers from homecare agencies understand how ALS affects the body. My purpose is to bring ALS out of the Dark Ages. It will be an extra bonus if it provides inspiration to all those afflicted with a terminal illness. These are the reasons I am writing this book.

When I was diagnosed with ALS in November of 1996, I knew only that it was a debilitating disease but had no clarity as to how it affects the body. ALS affects everyone differently. I have what is called bulbar, the worst type of ALS, which causes one to lose the ability to speak. As the disease progresses and the body becomes a wasteland of paralyzed muscles, patients are too weak to become vocal about their plight.

Family and caregivers are focused on around-the-clock care and are too emotionally drained to take up the cause for public awareness and funding. "Cries of the Silent" speaks for those who cannot speak, to those who have the compassion and desire to bring ALS out of the Dark Ages.

The reason that there is the level of awareness and funding for AIDS is that AIDS patients are able to be more vocal than ALS people.

By the time the ALS person wants to be vocal, the ability to speak is gone. The cause will have to be led by people who are caregivers or relatives who have gone through the experience, and you, the reader of this book. Life expectancy is two to five years, so there isn't a lot of time to be vocal.

The public is not aware of ALS and how little funding is available. Government funding for ALS was a mere $15,000 last year. This pales in comparison to AIDS funding, which is in the millions. In Canada, 1,000 people will be diagnosed with ALS this year, and two or three will die from it every day, compared to 640 people who contract AIDS every year.

This book is about my journey with ALS and my struggle to live my dying one day at a time. At the time of my diagnosis, I was determined that I would not be bitter. I would be better. It is a struggle every day not to give in to feelings of self-pity, especially when others reflect pity towards me.

I want to avoid entry into the dark hole of despair and depression. It is my desire to articulate my frustrations and challenges in the hope that this will give those who cannot   speak some hope or courage to carry on in their journey.

I speak with courage and conviction, but let me make it clear that it is not easy and I struggle with it every day, one day at a time. I do not think we master our feelings, but perhaps we can gain better control of them.

Since I was diagnosed with ALS, I have found that many people will not visit me because they are out of their comfort zone and either cannot deal with their feelings, or don't know how. Most people are uncomfortable with silence and don't know what to say. I hope this book will help them to become more aware and comfortable with ALS. Little do they know that just their presence is a comfort.

In my earlier reading, I learned that when diagnosed with a terminal illness, we go through four stages, which are denial, anger, grief and acceptance. I did not spend much time in the first two stages, but I did with grief, especially grieving the loss of my right hand, because I enjoyed communicating by writing letters, cards and sending faxes.

At this point, I am completely paralyzed and totally mute. I am able to communicate only when I sit in my recliner, wearing a special glass frame with a laser light attached to the side, which allows me to point the light to a spellboard in front of me.

Now that I have nearly completed the book, my neck has become so weak that pointing to each letter has become very strenuous. I find myself in tears grieving for what will ultimately happen when I am no longer able to hold my head up at all and lose all my ability to communicate. I know there will be many terrifying moments trying to communicate with only my eyes.

In this book, I have addressed the need to heal the whole body, not just physically, but intellectually, emotionally and spiritually. There is so much research on this subject that I wanted to delve into, but time and health would not permit. I have no doubt that my spirituality will carry me through to the end.

4

CHAPTER ONE

What is ALS?

Amyotrophic lateral sclerosis (ALS) is a progressive disease of the nervous system. The cause is not known and there is no cure, although progress is being made on both fronts. ALS is more commonly known as Lou Gehrig's disease, named after the famous baseball player who died from it.

ALS attacks motor neurons, which are among the largest of all nerve cells in the brain and spinal cord. These cells send messages to muscles throughout the body. With ALS, motor neurons die and the muscles do not receive these messages. As a result, muscles weaken as they lose their ability to move. Eventually, most muscle action is affected, including those which control swallowing and breathing, as well as major muscles in the arms, legs, back and neck. There is, however, no loss of sensory nerves, so people with ALS retain their sense of feeling, sight, hearing, smell and taste. The mind is not affected by this disease and people with ALS remain fully alert and aware of events.

The course of ALS is extremely variable and it is difficult to predict the rate of progression in any single patient. For the majority of people with ALS, weakness tends to progress over a three to five-year period.

ALS can strike anyone, at any age, but generally ALS occurs between the ages of forty and seventy. According to the National Institute of Health, some 4,600 people in the United States are newly diagnosed with ALS each year. Approximately four to six people per 100,000 worldwide get ALS. In a small percentage of patients, ALS is genetic.

What are the symptoms?

The first signs of ALS are often arm and leg weakness, muscle wasting and faint muscle rippling. These symptoms occur because muscles are no longer receiving the nutrient signals they need for growth and maintenance – a result of motor neurons dying. ALS nerve degeneration may also cause muscle cramps and vague pains, or problems with speech and swallowing. Some people with the disease may lose some control over their emotional responses. They laugh or cry much more easily than in the past. Eventually, all voluntary muscle action is affected.

How is ALS diagnosed?

There is no specific test for diagnosing ALS. However, several tests – including nerve conduction studies and electromyogram (EMG) – are used to measure how well and quickly the nerves are working. Ruling out other causes of muscular weakness is important because ALS often mimics other treatable diseases. Diagnosis requires special skills and neurological tests. People with ALS symptoms usually are referred to neurologists, who specialize in the nervous system. Diagnosis may take several months since an important part of the diagnostic process is to confirm disease progression.

What causes ALS?

The cause of ALS is unknown. It attacks its victims at random. However, it was recently discovered that five to ten percent of those with ALS show a definite genetic pattern. In this rare form, about one-half of the offspring may develop ALS. These people show a gene defect that affects an enzyme called superoxide dismutase. This enzyme eliminates toxic substances called free radicals. Free radicals can cause nerve cells to die and are associated with a number of diseases and even implicated in aging itself. For most people with ALS, the vast majority of their children are not at any greater risk of developing this disease than the general population. This type of ALS is often called "sporadic ALS" due to its unpredictable nature.

ALS researchers have found no difference between the symptoms and disease progression in the sporadic and genetic forms of ALS. Therefore, since the genetic and acquired forms of ALS appear to be similar, an understanding of the cause of the genetic form could lead to treatment for all forms of the disease.

Treatment

While there is no cure for ALS, research to solve the ALS puzzle is ongoing. Scientific advances have led to approval of the first treatment for the disease – a medication that may increase survival time. Other treatments under investigation include several nerve growth factors, which may help maintain quality of life by maintaining nerve function. While each of these therapies represent a step forward for people with ALS, a cure remains to be discovered.

For the majority of people with ALS, the primary treatment remains the management of ALS symptoms. Patients need to take an active role in the design of their treatment regimen. Ideally, ALS management involves physical, occupational, speech, respiratory and nutrition therapy. For instance, certain drugs and the application of heat or whirlpool therapy may help to relieve muscle cramping. Exercise can help maintain muscle strength and function. Exercise, however, is recommended in moderation. Drugs also may be used to help combat fatigue, but in some patients may worsen muscle cramps.

As the disease progresses, various assistive devices will help persons with ALS maintain their independence and ensure personal safety. For example, an ankle/foot brace can improve function and conserve energy, as well as help avoid injury. When neck, trunk and shoulder weakness makes walking or sitting difficult, cervical collars, perhaps with an additional chest and head strap, provide helpful support. A reclining chair is preferable to a headrest to relieve fatigue of neck muscles. There are also numerous devices to assist in feeding, dressing and maintaining personal hygiene. Eventually, more substantial equipment, such as wheelchairs, scooters, lifts and hospital beds may be required.

It is important to know that speech therapists can help with speech and swallowing difficulties as they develop. Also, drug treatments can help patients who develop excessive saliva and drooling.

Family members of people with ALS should be instructed in the Heimlich maneuver to provide assistance in a life-threatening choking episode. Feeding tubes may be necessary to maintain nutrition, as may breathing devices when the disease affects the muscles of the chest. However, with these supportive devices, there are physical, emotional and financial implications, and their use should be discussed with a physician well in advance of when the need arises. Managing the symptoms is a process that is challenging for people with ALS, their caregivers, and their medical team.

Of all the disabilities that affect a person with ALS, one of the most devastating and most common is the progressive loss of the ability to communicate. However, advances in computer technology mean that persons with ALS today have vital new electronic communications options that can be adapted to their individual capabilities.

Progress through research

Significant progress is being made in the study of ALS. Although there is still no cure, recent clinical trials have shown that some drugs affect nerve cell activity and may increase the survival time for people with ALS. Newly developed animal models of the genetic form of the disease, so-called transgenic ALS mice, offer neurologic researchers the ability to test therapies in mice. There is great hope that this and other neuroscientific advances will lead to a cure in humans. Talk with your doctor about being involved in future clinical trials or about the drugs currently available for the treatment of this disease.

CHAPTER TWO

My Fifty Years

On April 17, 1996 my family and friends gathered at our home for a surprise birthday celebration for my big 50th. It was fun times with flowers and gifts. The usual jokes about aging were flowing freely. I remember making a comment about having difficulty holding on to my wineglass with my left hand. My sister Laura jokingly responded that that's what happens when you have had too much wine. I didn't realize at the time that this observation of my left hand would impact my entire life.

As I looked down memory lane, browsing through photo albums, I reflected on my fifty years of life. I thought of what a happy childhood I'd had.

I grew up on a farm near a little village town called Primate, in Saskatchewan. I was the eldest in a family of five girls and two boys. My parents offered us all the physical, emotional, intellectual and spiritual nourishment that they were capable of providing for us.

My parents worked very hard to make a living growing wheat and raising cattle. I can still see my father walking at a fast clip across the farmyard. He was a successful farmer who was always on top of things. My mother not only managed the household, but also helped in the fields and performed other farm chores. As we grew up, we all shared in responsibilities, both indoors and out.

My first few years of school, I walked or travelled by horse and buggy to the school which was about 2 miles away. When I reached junior high we had the luxury of a school bus that picked us up in our yard. Arriving home from school we could smell Mom's home baking before we even entered the house. We always had good food and home made clothes. Sometimes Mom would dress all the girls in the same outfit. She was a great seamstress and we would pick out a dress we liked in the Eaton's or Sears catalogue and she would cut the pattern out of paper to make it. We were indeed the envy of our friends. In the winter months, I would stay with my grandparents in town. I enjoyed life in town more than the country because I could visit friends any-time. Those were the early signs of being a social butterfly.

In Grade 11, I attended a private school, St. Angela's Academy in Prelate, Saskatchewan. There I took thirteen subjects and had excellent grades, perhaps because there were no male distractions. It was a time for spiritual growth, which I am grateful for.

In Grade 12 I met a young man at a dance who would be my future husband. I knew of him from provincial track and field competitions because we both competed for our respective schools. His name was Larry Bell and he was in his second year of university.

I went to Saskatoon Business College for two years while Larry finished his degree in Education. There we both developed many lasting friendships.

In 1967 we moved to Calgary. I like to say that I moved to Calgary first and Larry followed me. He would have his own version of the story. In November of that year we were married.

Larry taught at Vincent Massey Junior High School and I worked in the Physical Education Department for the Calgary Public School Board. A year later I worked for Dr. Lionel McLeod in the Internal Medicine Department at the Foothills Hospital. In 1970 we had our first son, Derek. He had a great disposition, which he still has today. I enjoyed motherhood very much and decided on a job that would keep me at home. I bought a fifty-dollar skin care kit from Nutri-Metics International and would do in-home presentations at night when Larry was home. I had never sold anything in my life, but I was surprised at how well the sales went. I soon realized that I was not just selling products but I was also selling a feeling of well being. I could not believe how many women would focus on their negative features rather than the positive ones.

In 1972 we were blessed with our second son, Jarret. He was a delightful baby and motherhood was most fulfilling. The thought of putting the boys in daycare was enough to motivate me to continue on with my small Nutri-Metics business.

In 1977 Larry quit teaching to go into partnership with two other friends to build squash and racquetball courts. In 1978 our third son, Travis was born. The business turned out to be a bad decision and we lost a lot of money and valuable family time. We worked long hours before we sold it at a great loss. This experience tested our marriage and financial security.

We knew that we could always replace money but not our health or our marriage. Life for us went on at a feverish pace. Larry went back to teaching after selling the club. It was a challenge to juggle homemaking, parenting, business, gardening, interior decorating and chauffeuring, but I loved the roles and performed them with great intensity.

Travis brought the family great joy. At age three, we almost lost him when he developed epiglotitis. He was in an oxygen tent for a few days and it was a traumatic experience for us all.

As the years sped away, the boys became ever so independent. The teen years brought some new challenges that we had to rise to. They were heavily involved in sports during every season. Larry was their personal coach while I cheered from the sidelines.

Just like their parents, our sons were very athletic and it was a joy to see them perform in soccer, softball, basketball, football and hockey. Graduation was here before we were ready for it. Today we still hear stories about mischievous times that we were unaware of when they happened.

On September 25, 1992, our family suffered a great loss, when my father died of cancer of the liver.

At the time of his diagnosis, he was told he had only a few days to live. This came as a terrible shock to us all and I didn't realize at the time that I was in a state of depression for a few months after my father's death. The family pulled together to support my mother and we all made more frequent visits home to Provost to spend time with her.

Sundays were and still are family days with special dinners and pleasant conversation. Often friends or extended family would be invited to join us and the boys would invite their girl friends.

Our sons took their time deciding on their careers. In 1997, Derek married Christy, a wonderful lady, who is beautiful both inside and out. She had a five-year-old daughter, Jasmine, who is delightful and brings us much joy.

During the years of raising a family, my Nutri-Metics business grew extensively and I enjoyed many company cars and numerous trips to foreign lands. I reached many levels of success in the business, being top achiever in Canada for a number of years. I felt I wanted to be a success at parenting and everything I did, so my business did not get my undivided attention. I learned a great deal about human behavior while creating an environment for people to be the best they could and to help them establish their own independent businesses.

I would soak up all the information in self-help books and belonged to Achievers Canada, through which I was privileged to hear many professional speakers. This prepared me for what was to come.

On May 24, 1998 our first grandson, Isaiah was born. It was three weeks later that Derek and Christy brought him home to us. He was and is absolutely gorgeous. The most painful thing was not being able to hold or kiss him. Derek would lay him on my lap or beside my face in bed. That way I could hear his heart beat and smell him.

I looked on with great pride as I saw what wonderful parents Derek and Christy had become. It was always difficult to say good-bye when they left for their home in Edgewood, B.C.

Jarret is in his last year of University as I write this in September 1998. He will graduate in Outdoor Pursuits in spring of '99. He has been a student for six years and is anxious to start his own business in the great outdoors. Travis left home at age sixteen to play hockey in Victoria, B.C., where he also finished Grade 12. It was difficult to let him go at the time, but we recognized the opportunity for a hockey scholarship and character building.

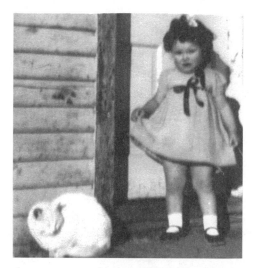

2 years old

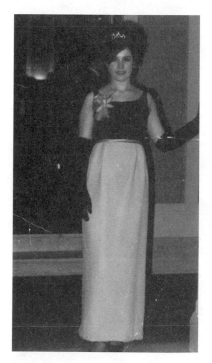

College Queen

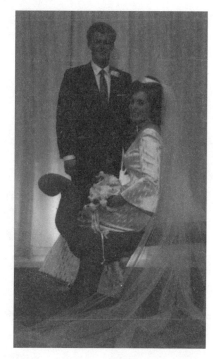

Wedding Day

14

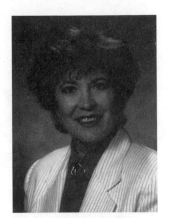

49 years old

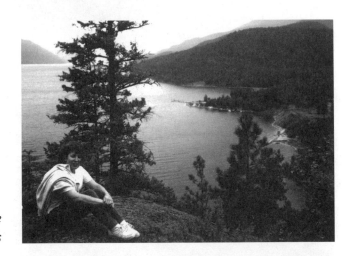

*Summer before
diagnosis*

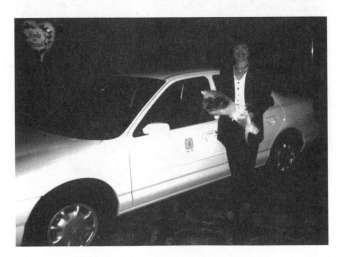

*Presentation of
Nutri Metics Car*

CHAPTER THREE

Three Diagnoses

In the spring of 1996 I became aware of clumsiness in my left hand. I would notice it when buttoning clothes, picking weeds or cutting food. I also experienced unusual fatigue.

I went to a chiropractor, thinking it was a pinched nerve. I also saw my family doctor who had no explanation for my symptoms, but set up an appointment for me to see a neurologist who ruled out a brain tumor. I then saw him a second time and he said he was stumped as to what I had. He then referred me to another neurologist but my appointments kept getting postponed for no apparent reason. Finally on November 2, 1996 I saw the second neurologist. He examined me briefly and then called me to his office. After taking a brief family history, he dropped the bomb!

It was a very traumatic experience. The room was stark and devoid of warmth. He sat behind his desk in a white uniform, showing no emotion and said "What you have is ALS". I asked, "What is that"? He replied, "It is better known as Lou Gehrig's disease". I asked him if that was what Sue Rodrigues had and he said, "yes". Then I lost it. I was in total shock and disbelief.

He pushed a box of Kleenex toward me and asked if he could bring in an assistant. He introduced her as an intern. My world turned upside-down and I could not think clearly. He mentioned that there was no known cause or cure for ALS. I asked what my prognosis was and he replied "three years", still not showing any emotion.

He mentioned something about drugs, but I didn't hear anymore, still trying to comprehend my death sentence. He asked if I had a ride home. I said I came to the appointment alone, thinking it was just an examination. I wished Larry had been there. I wished the doctor had held me and shown some compassion and empathy. I left to find my car in the parking lot. Driving home was a real challenge, trying to see through the blur of tears.

When I arrived home I told Larry about my diagnosis and was surprised that he didn't lose it. He told me that after talking to a friend, Don Norman, he had suspected that I could have ALS. Don's wife, Betty was diagnosed with ALS in August of that same year. The hardest thing would be – how do we tell our sons? We decided to tell our brothers and sisters first to have a support system in place for our parents. We phoned Jarret and asked him to come over. When we told him, he was very calm and said that he also suspected something serious pertaining to the nervous system, because he had learned about motor neurons in his kinesiology classes. He said he had already cried many times and had prepared himself. We said we would stay positive and beat this disease.

When we phoned Derek and Christy and broke the news, Derek was silent, and after asking some questions, he sobbed. We wished we could have been there to hug him and I asked Christy to be strong for him. They said they would make a trip home shortly.

We debated about how much to tell Travis, who was sixteen at the time. It was a short debate because we both knew he would go to the library and check it out. When we phoned him he was excited about all the things that were happening in his life with hockey. It was heart breaking to tell him the news.

He reacted with sobs and lots of questions. We made arrangements to fly him home. That following weekend we were all together and tried to come to grips with what would change our lives dramatically. We read everything we could find on ALS.

I would wake up at night and think I had just had a bad dream. When morning came I would think about how independent I was and how I soon would become totally dependent on my loved ones. All sorts of fearful thoughts entered my mind about the journey with ALS, but not the destination. I was not angry with God. I recognized it as my new mission. Life is a gift and I trusted in God and His divine plan.

I went back to see the doctor to request a second opinion and to ask if he would make an appointment with a neurologist in Edmonton. He said he would but that would not change the diagnosis. Arrangements were made for me to fly up for another neurological assessment in January.

Christmas was sad for me as I wondered whether it would be the last one with my family. We hosted that Christmas with our extended family. The love and support that surrounded me was heart warming.

When January came, my sister Vel picked me up at the airport. We headed straight for the hospital to have an MRI and strength test done before I would meet with the doctor. The neurologist performed the same brief examination that had been done on me before and then said, "I don't think you have ALS". I could not believe that I had heard right, so I asked him to repeat himself. "What you have is called Focal Motor Neuron Disease, which focuses on just one limb". With that I fell back on the examining table in disbelief. Vel and I looked at each other with great anticipation. The doctor went on to say that he recognized it because a friend of his had been diagnosed with FMND some years ago. He said to come back in ten years and see his associate because he would be retired by then.

The new diagnosis that it wasn't terminal and only would affect my left arm was exhilarating. I said, "I can handle a gimpy arm". I still had one concern that I wanted him to address. I mentioned that I noticed a difference in my handwriting in that it was messy and felt awkward. I wrote with my right hand. He then called in an associate to do some strength tests on both hands. He did not seem too concerned about that. He left the room and my sister and I hugged each other.

My girlfriend, Shirley Speers had been waiting outside. We called her in and she was elated with the good news. I said I was buying lunch and we would celebrate with wine. We had a fun-filled and leisurely lunch. I said I didn't need a plane, that I could fly home on my own.

When I arrived in Calgary, Larry was upset about the plane's arrival time. He was muttering to himself. I said "Forget about the damn plane, I don't have ALS!" He looked at me in disbelief and asked me what I meant. We hugged. Words cannot express our joy.

We could not wait to break the good news to the boys and our families. Everyone was overjoyed.

A week later, we left for Club Med in Mexico. My company had a seminar there and I was a featured speaker. All my colleagues from Canada and the U.S. were happy about the good news. That week I spent a lot of time in my room, feeling very fatigued. I thought it was from the roller coaster high I had just experienced. Others thought likewise. The surroundings were breathtaking and the ocean waves soothing. It was definitely the best environment to unwind and rejuvenate.

I began to recognize the same symptoms that occurred in my left hand were now manifesting in my right hand. I also noticed some difficulty in speaking. This was not supposed to happen with Focal Motor Neuron Disease.

I made another appointment with the neurologist in Edmonton for the end of March. When I saw him, I knew that he knew that I had ALS. He apologized for the wrong diagnosis. I wasn't angry with him because I valued the two months of freedom. He explained the drugs for which I would be a selected candidate. I said I wanted all the information on them and would discuss it with my husband.

This time it was more difficult to go through the steps of recovery. First is anger, then grieving and finally acceptance and healing. These were the steps that our family had to go through as well. This was a roller coaster ride. My heart went out to Larry and the boys.

I proceeded once again to bury myself in books about healing and got strength in reading the bible. I continued listening to relaxation tapes and doing meditation. Water aerobics became more difficult now with both hands going limp. I started yoga, which dealt with body, mind and soul. There were things that I could not do but I wouldn't let that discourage me. I checked out acupuncture and decided to take ten treatments. This also included brain entrainment with the use of lights and music, which were to build new pathways of thinking. I found them to be very relaxing and meditative.

One doctor I saw questioned whether or not I knew about amalgam fillings. I had read about that and yes, I had several. I was very disappointed in this doctor because all he was interested in was selling me vitamins. What made it worse was the $100.00 cover charge and no satisfaction. I asked the neurologist about amalgam fillings and he said there was no evidence to support the theory that they may cause neurological damage. I questioned if the fillings were replaced, what about leakage of mercury. He shrugged his shoulders.

I was not interested in the drugs that were available to me. There were too many risks or side effects and I would rather have quality of life than feel nauseous, fatigued and listless. There were no guarantees that the drugs would be effective and they were still in the early phase of experimentation. I did agree to be involved in research for MRI and strength tests every month. Thanks to the businesses that donated air miles to muscular dystrophy that enabled me to fly free to Edmonton each month for the tests.

Once a month I would go to the ALS clinic to see specialists and be assessed. I never did go to the monthly ALS support group meetings as I felt that I did not want to expose myself to feelings of despair. I felt strong emotionally, but perhaps not strong enough to uplift others. There would be a time when I would be able to provide comfort and support to others afflicted with ALS, but not at that point.

In June of 1997 we moved to a bungalow that would be more wheelchair accessible than our two-story home. By the end of June I had to give up driving because turning corners became more challenging. In July I retired from my business. I received many cards and letters from my clients and peers, which were very gratifying.

Derek announced he was getting married on August 2nd, which would be in three weeks. It would be a small wedding on the acreage where they lived in Edgewood, B.C. I had nightmares about not being prepared, but Derek and Christy assured us that all would be looked after. People pull together in small communities.

The celebration turned out fine and all details were taken care of. We gained a beautiful daughter, Christy, as well as her daughter, Jasmine. Everyone enjoyed the outdoor wedding. The day was sunny and the surroundings of trees and hills were like a chapel. It was a wonderful day for both families as well as friends.

A week later, my sister, Laura got married, which was another great family celebration. Although my left leg was stiff, I managed to have a dance with Larry and Travis.

After the wedding, all my sisters and brothers met at my mother's house in Provost, Alberta. Mom had made the decision to sell her house and move in with us to help with meals and caregiving. She gave away all her furniture and belongings to her children. Everyone took what they wanted and moved it to their respective homes. This way, mom would feel at home wherever she went. It was a relief to have her move in with us because Larry had to go back to work after summer vacation and it was a challenge for me to prepare meals.

The fall of 1997 brought more changes in my health. I wrote a paper on "A Day with ALS" to create awareness.

A Day with ALS

Our bodies are not made to last forever on this earth, but imagine waking up one morning and this is your reality.

You are faced with a diagnosis of a fatal disease. ALS – possibly two to five years to live; dealing with the daily and future challenges of the slow ravages of this disease; daily diminution of your bodily functions as you prepare for death. It sounds like an emotion packed movie or a bad dream, doesn't it? Slowly the reality hits you – all the things you could do independently are now a memory. The every day world, the way you knew it, will never be the same. Your mind and emotions are racing uncontrollably like a yo-yo until you rationally try to come to terms with your condition.

Come with me on a daily journey. It's time to get up, your mouth is parched and dry and you can't talk. The weakening facial muscles cause you to sleep with your mouth open; therefore, you need water before you can even utter the softest sound. Hopefully, you have a loving spouse, like I do, to help you. Your desire is to jump out of bed to relieve all the pressure points and sore joints of your body, but of course, you can't!

You try to roll on your side, but you can't. Your left hand and arm won't move; your right arm and shoulder are weak and extremely painful because you slept too long on one side. You try to lift your legs, but energy is in short supply there also. You definitely need someone to pivot you out of bed so that you can start your day. But before that can happen, you'll need physio to eliminate the stiffness and, hopefully, maintain some range of motion of your limbs. Thank God for your marvelous spouse, aided by the home care person.

In 1993, I experienced burnout and fatigue but it wasn't like the profound fatigue you have with ALS. Therefore, you must practice conserving energy on a daily basis if you are afflicted with ALS.

For a clear analogy, let's say a healthy person has $500.00 worth of energy to expend each day. With ALS you would perhaps have $100.00. The wasted muscles feel like you are carrying dead weights in each limb. This is an approximation of how you spend your energy:

- *Walking (with assistance up until Feb. '98) - $10*
- *Morning and evening routine (dressing, washing, etc.) - $20*
- *Meals (three or four) - $30*
- *Trying to talk (up until Jan. '98) - $10*
- *Writing (up until March '98) - $5*
- *Bathing and hair care - $20*
- *Transfers from wheelchair - $10*
- *Total - $100 all spent*

When the above activities are carried out without frustration, the amount of energy spent is half of $100.

The energy drain is most severe when anxiety and frustration exist. These energy drains occur when caregivers are focused on their own thoughts instead of what they are doing, or what they are forgetting. Energy is restored with good nutrition (thanks to my dear mother), rest and a positive environment.

Every day you decide how you will "parcel out" your $100 worth of energy; therefore, you learn to pace yourself. You however, get very tired of being constantly tired.

The most frustrating part of this type of ALS (Bulbar) is not being able, as the disease advances, to speak or communicate your basic needs. How much you would like to shed light on the many false assumptions or misunderstandings. How dearly you desire to communicate so that you can acknowledge people around you – what they say and do, give and send. Your listening skills are very astute and you hear and sense things about family, friends and visitors that they themselves don't realize. It feels like living on an island all by yourself. Being housebound, your link to the world is in cards, letters, faxes, television and books.

Your intellect is spared with ALS, everything seems clearer than before or perhaps you have more time for reflection! Also, your senses of sight, sound, taste, smell and feeling are intact. How nice it would be to chomp on crunchy food instead of pureed. At this point in time, I can only swallow, not chew. The next step will be a feeding tube.

How one handles ALS emotionally is One Day at a Time. I get my strength from God. It is difficult to control one's emotions. It is difficult because I cannot hold back the physical tears due to wasted facial muscles and extreme fatigue. Tears fall easily as ALS patients want to express themselves emotionally, i.e. greetings or good-byes or after exhausting oneself to communicate unsuccessfully. The most difficult thing emotionally is not being able to kiss loved ones.

Visitors and others comment on how good you look and how misleading this can be because it has no relevance to how you are physically. Physically, I look very thin because of wasted muscles. The motor neurons die. The muscles are wasted and paralyzed. Every month you notice further weakness and muscle deterioration.

The following are some of the daily physical challenges and dis-comforts:

- *daily communication – regarding food, needs or an itch*
- *can't blow nose or drain saliva*
- *trying to move food around in the mouth with a paralyzed tongue and dropped palette*
- *morsels of food stuck under tongue and in gums*
- *food leaks out of mouth due to inability to press lips together firmly*
- *unable to walk to attend to bathroom needs or stretch stiff limbs without assistance*
- *unable to turn the pages when I love to read*
- *unable to lift head forward when it falls back*
- *unable to use hands except to laboriously scribble this*
- *total dependence on others*

Spiritually, you can rise as you turn to God and accept a Divine Plan – not, of course, necessarily understood. I find developing a strong relationship with our Lord helps to focus on eternity rather than the things of this world. Also, placing my faith and trust in God for the things we have no control over. Before the eternal hello, it is important to live our dying. So, I try to live each day to the fullest. I give thanks to God for three or four things or people everyday, which keeps my perspective on life. I try not to focus on the things that are missing.

I am blessed to have three sons and a daughter-in-law, a spouse and mother who shower me with love, in their thoughts, words and deeds. I am also fortunate to have a loving extended family and relatives and friends. This is such a good support and helps get me through the rough spots.

"A Day with ALS" has been written to create a greater awareness about how ALS affects the body and how one copes with this relentless disease. It is my hope that people will have a better understanding and courage to talk and ask questions about ALS.

Some people see the disease and not the person and keep their distance. This is painful for both them and me, however, I understand. I am still the same person.

This disease is approximately 130 years old. It is so disheartening that researchers have not found the cause of, or the cure for this mysterious disease. Hopefully, everyone's efforts and contributions toward fundraising for research will help find a cure or offer a better quality of life for others who may get ALS.

to be continued. . . . . .

Written by Evelyn Bell with a laser light attached to her glasses, using a spellboard, while a friend writes.

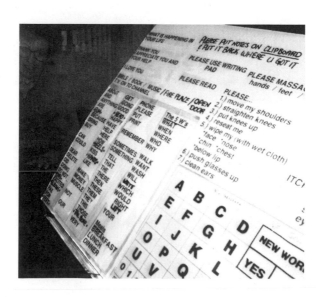

WHY COMPLAIN

Why whine and complain?

*When the words and thoughts are verbalized the damage
has begun*

It manifests itself in your body in some way

High blood pressure - headache or heartache

It takes away your power to be in control of the situation

It magnifies the problem

It reduces the energy level

The choice is clear, become bitter or better

Evelyn Bell

CHAPTER FOUR

Succumb or Overcome

When we made the dreaded phone calls to the family about my affliction, I decided I would not become bitter. I would choose to become better. There is always hope, because without hope, what is there? I did not want to be drawn into the dark hole of despair, knowing I would not be happy there and I didn't want to chase people away. I enjoyed the many visitors who took my mind off myself. I recognized my affliction as a mission, trusting in God that there was a greater understanding in the human link of the Divine plan.

We all have fears about death.

Why is everyone so afraid of death? Could it be that we are afraid to lose our power, our identity, our ego, and our future? Our future is temporary on earth but everlasting in the Kingdom of God. For me, it is more the departure from my family and not being there for them when they are raising families of their own that I fear. Grandchildren are a blessing, and how I would love to spend time with them. But who knows what heaven has in store.

The more familiar we become with God's word, the less fear of death we will have. I take comfort in the following passage from ll Corinthians 5:1-8:

For we know that when this earthly tent we live in is taken down - when we die and leave these bodies – we will have a home in heaven, an eternal body made for us by God himself and not by human hands. We grow weary in our present bodies and we long for the day when we will put on our heavenly bodies like new clothing. For we will not be spirits without bodies. Our dying bodies make us groan and sigh, but it's not that we want to die and have no bodies at all. We want to slip into our new bodies so that these dying bodies will be swallowed up by everlasting life. God himself has prepared us for this and as a guarantee he has given us his Holy Spirit.

So we are always confident, even though we know that as long as we live in these bodies, we are not at home with the Lord. That is why we live by believing and not by seeing. Yes, we are fully confident, and we would rather be away from these bodies, for then we will be at home with the Lord.

In life we are always in pursuit of happiness. I would define happiness as an event like opening a Christmas gift, travelling places or purchasing new things, but this happiness does not last. We work feverishly for the natural things of this world, but it is never enough.

I have found, since being diagnosed with this disease, that looking inward and upward more toward the Kingdom of God is where true joy abides. This joy is lasting and not elusive, like happiness. I believe that those of us who are afflicted with physical, emotional or spiritual pain can find joy if we choose to.

As the disease progresses and the muscles waste away, it is difficult not to grieve for what you no longer have. I can no longer walk or talk. Both my arms and hands are totally paralyzed. I can't even move one finger voluntarily. My choice of food is very limited because I can only swallow it whole. I am unable to chew because my tongue is paralyzed, which makes it impossible to roll the food in my mouth and move it around my gums or between my teeth. My neck is weak and my head often falls forward.

Fortunately I can turn my head from side to side while using a laser light attached to my glasses. As I point to each letter, a friend types up the sentences that will go into this book. It is very tedious, but I am determined to finish it. My neck is getting weaker, but if I do this in the morning, I find that I have more energy to point to the correct letters. I would not be able to write this book without the dedication of friends who volunteer their time each day.

Sometimes nights seem to last forever. Sleeping is a challenge because I can't turn, move any limbs, or roll from one side to another to relieve pressure points. I sleep on my back most of the time and Larry or a caregiver turns me to my side once during the night. If I yawn or have a muscle spasm, my hands will move out of place and I have to wake one of them up to make adjustments to my body. On a good night, I will need three adjustments, but a bad night could mean as many as twelve adjustments. We now have a caregiver every other night, which allows Larry to get his rest. If I have a choking spell, my hands and feet need to be adjusted. Sometimes my whole body has to be reseated in the wheelchair. With each swallow, my head goes down for ease of swallowing. Sometimes food runs out of my mouth when my head drops forward.

It is messy because my tongue is paralyzed and cannot move the food to the back of my mouth. I prefer to eat with only the caregiver because it requires concentration on both of our parts.

I used to take multi vitamins and antioxidants, but I can't now. I get my nutrients in a drink called Jevity, which is all I need. I have four of these drinks through my stomach tube every day, along with clear juices and water. Eating and drinking require a lot of energy.

After breakfast I get washed and have my teeth brushed. The challenge in brushing my teeth is to keep my mouth open. Sometimes it involuntarily shuts and I clamp down on the toothbrush. I cannot gargle or hold my head back to rinse and I swallow more toothpaste than I want to.

Face creams are applied every morning and night to soothe the dryness caused from so much wiping with tissues. There is constant wiping of my mouth because I cannot swallow much saliva. There is a lot of discomfort in drooling and having my mouth wiped. Some will wipe my mouth and spread the saliva all over my chin and cheeks. This too requires a skill to wipe from the outside corners to the center of my lips. Sometimes I get my mouth and nose wiped together. All this requires a lot of my patience.

My mom and I watch and participate in a televised mass every morning at 9:00 A.M.. This is a great way to start my day with the Lord. About 10:00 A.M. one of several friends who volunteer arrives to scribe while I point to the letters on the spellboard. We do this for one to two hours, depending on my energy level. We usually complete a page or two for the book. I feel very fortunate and blessed to have these five friends and my niece who volunteer their time for two hours every day.

At 11:00 every morning I have two cans of Jevity because I do not eat lunch orally. I will have one can at 4:00 P.M. and two more cans for dinner. Often I am even too tired to eat four spoonfuls at dinner. At noon I go for a two-hour nap. My caregiver, Bruce Mitchell, puts me to bed and gives me my physio after I wake up. We have our challenging moments communicating. Bruce is a very positive person with a keen sense of humor and lots of energy. His humor matches mine so we get along great.

If I did not have physio or range of motion work everyday, I would have curled hands, feet and probably would not stand so well. I still have strength in my legs, especially the right one. If all the steps are followed for transferring me, I will snap out of my wheelchair or recliner with no difficulty, but if some steps are forgotten, I cannot bear weight. Sometimes caregivers, including family, are in a trance of their own and this is when I will be put into a state of discomfort. When you work with someone who can't speak, caregivers need to be on the ball at all times.

At 4:00 P.M. each day I enjoy Oprah. Her show is usually inspirational and informative and sometimes very moving. She is a powerful lady because she influences millions in a positive way. I wish there were more shows like hers. I watch very little television because I don't want a passive mind. So much on TV is mindless and requires viewer discretion. I watch the news to keep up with what's happening in the world, but I do not read the newspaper because there is too much negative news regarding crime.

In the evening if we don't have company, my husband and I will visit briefly with the spellboard or we will watch something humorous on television. By 9:00 P.M. I am very tired and ready for bed. My sister Sandy and sister-in-law Lynda each come over one night a week to help Larry prepare me for bed.

Once I am in bed, it is a challenge for family and caregivers to get all my limbs, back, neck and head positioned where I am comfortable. When I cough, yawn or have a muscle spasm everything needs to be readjusted. This can happen several times a night.

Sometimes during the night I have to be turned over onto my

side to prevent bedsores from developing. This procedure is very challenging for both caregivers and me because everything has to be precise or my legs will straighten out and my spine will not be supported. Sometimes I do not get a good sleep because of pressure points on my butt, hands, heels and ankles. The pain caused by these pressure points is like a constant gnawing.

My body feels like it is entrenched in clay. I can't move my upper body at all. I can move my legs up and down but not from side to side. My mouth gets very dry from breathing with my mouth open. Caregivers will give me water from a bottle and drip drops into my mouth while I'm sleeping. Sometimes they spill on my neck, which wakes me up. It is always a challenge for both caregivers and me when communicating what I need adjusted in bed. We go through a process of elimination, as they mention each limb.

Anxiety is my constant companion. My muscles tense up when I need to remind caregivers about what they miss seeing, when it seems so obvious to me. Things like leaning to one side or the other in the recliner or the wheelchair, a wet nose, chin, lips or a hair in my face.

Some patients with ALS lose control over their emotional responses. I am one of them. There is no muscle control when it comes to holding back the tears. Tears fall easily when I haven't seen someone in a while or something touches me deeply. Tears also fall often when in distress or frustrated.

The thing that frustrates me the most is when I am put in a state of discomfort, because caregivers are distracted with their own thoughts instead of what they are doing with me. This happens daily and I try not to respond with tears, but it is impossible.

Perhaps I am expecting too much. We can only focus on one thing at a time and I realize that caregivers care for more than one patient in a day. Often they will transfer me like any other patient but that doesn't work for me. Some days numerous things are forgotten, which heightens my anxiety and I try to mumble to alert them, but to no avail.

When this happens, I say a prayer, or if it happens repeatedly, I cry in frustration. Later I will write about what transpired and why I was upset. I request that they review the carebook, but I know for some it is only read one time, which explains why there is so much forgotten.

When I refer to caregivers, I am referring to family as well. I say this, not to criticize, but to create awareness. I feel that there should be special training for caregivers who care for those that are mute, to reduce frustration for both caregiver and patient. Perhaps one day there will be an agency that will specialize in caregiving for ALS patients, especially those that can not communicate vocally.

We have had to replace two caregivers because of their health. We then go through the process of advertising and alerting agencies to help find a good replacement. My husband and I interview prospects and request references. Then comes the training, which is very challenging and tiring for both of us. During this training period, I find myself exhausted and short of breath. It takes about six weeks for things to go smoothly and for the caregiver to read my eyes and gestures.

The four caregivers that we now have are very compassionate, patient and dedicated. They are punctual and can be counted on to always be on the job. We are fond of each one of them.

I am committed to being my own best caregiver. By that I mean that I will always make an effort to co-operate with caregivers. I envision the hand of the Lord reaching out to help me when family and caregivers assist me.

If I were asked what my coping skills were, I would respond with the following:

1. Have an unbridled faith in God. Ask for guidance in building a relationship with God. Pray and reflect daily and ask for strength in my journey.

2. Show gratitude for the blessings in my life, everyday. I am grateful for what I have to work with rather than focusing on my handicaps. I am grateful for my intellect, senses and my humor, for family, friends, caregivers, the comforts of home and the love that surrounds me. There are so many things that one can be grateful for everyday.

3. Have a purpose. My purpose has been to inspire others with how I deal with my afflictions rather than turn them away with self-pity and bitterness. Also, my purpose is to create awareness about the need for research and equipment for ALS patients.

5. Have a commitment to a higher goal. I focus on the heavenly

kingdom – not the earthly goals.

1 Corinthians: 2.9
No eye has seen, no ear has heard, and no mind has imagined what God has prepared for those who love Him.

6. Squeeze as much out of life as I can by living in the moment and one day at a time.

7. Realize that I am not the only one with ALS or some other terminal illness, and that everyone's life is limited.

9. See the positive in living and dying. I try to live my dying.

11. See the humor in things. Laughter is such good medicine.

12. Embrace ALS when it progresses and when it becomes overwhelming. Embrace it on all levels, physically, emotionally, intellectually and spiritually.

13. Do not allow anyone to make you feel that you are a burden. (A priest gave me this advice).

YESTERDAY I CRIED

Yesterday I cried and cried
'Til my eyes were swollen and red.
I did not want to hear that I had a fatal disease.
No known cause or cure.
There was so much I wanted to do.

Yesterday I cried when I felt that familiar twitch
Invading my muscles.
I recognized that ALS was on the move.

Yesterday I cried when I saw my skeleton body
In the mirror.
My back feels like a washboard
When caregivers rub lotion on my skin.

Yesterday I cried when I could no longer walk
Or run in the park.
When I could no longer eat or prepare my family's favourite meals;
When I could no longer speak to my loved ones,
Or talk to friends on the phone.

Yesterday I cried when I could no longer make love to my husband;
When I could no longer hug or kiss my loved ones;
When I could no longer go on a holiday.

Yesterday I cried when I could no longer write letters or faxes;
When I could no longer read my bible or books.

Yesterday I cried tears of frustration for the daily misunderstandings;
Perceptions can be so varied.

Yesterday I cried tears of joy and gratitude for the people
Who lovingly take care of me every day and night;
For all the volunteers who give so generously of their time;
For Almighty God who is my refuge, strength and stronghold.

Evelyn Bell

CHAPTER FIVE

Frustrations & Challenges

There is a lot I have lost in my body since the onset of this disease. I am writing this in September 1998, now totally dependent on my family and caregivers. Reading my journal, I realize I have come a distance since November 1996. The following excerpts will reveal the emotional struggles and how I have dealt with them...

Journal entries commencing March, 1997

Today I want to turn loose old hurts, stop dwelling on the past (i.e. wrong diagnosis, lack of care and concern by doctors, grieving for lost left limb). I want to convert my "reactions" to pleasant ones. Oh God, help me to alter my attitude and change my life. I take up my cross and follow you. Have mercy upon me and save me from trying to find "excuses". Amen

Is it possible to turn those negative emotions that disturb my "comfort zone" into positive sources of energy? Contentment comes from the capacity to reprogram ourselves and experience a kind of "conversion" whereby we learn to be willing to be uncomfortable. One way, of course is to begin to look upon distressing conditions as "normal" or anticipated. I will no longer worry about the stress of anger, fear or anxiety, but become somewhat immune to their impact upon me. Could I expand my comfort zone to the point that I make it possible for me to be comfortable being uncomfortable? I will have to learn to manage all kinds of circumstances, challeng-

ing my right limb, which I am grateful for. Also, grateful for the gift of LIFE and good health. I'm grateful that my mother, husband, children and extended families have good health.

"How I see my affliction"

I have never thought of this health challenge as "Why me Lord?" or "What did I do to deserve this?" Nor have I felt anger towards God. But rather I immediately recognized it as a mission. "What is it I am to do in my life?" What is my job on earth? I saw it as a wake-up call, a challenge to re-direct my life; change my circumstances about my job. It still is a journey of self-discovery to make inner changes that are necessary for me to become a healed person. This will require life-strife changes to some degree. And more than anything, it has called attention to a greater spiritual awareness. I want to understand life at a higher level and I pray for God's guidance and direction in my life on earth. The trials of my left limb have something to teach me.

In looking at physical diseases, traditional medicine/doctors tend to concentrate on the body and act as though a person, mind and soul do not come with it. But they cannot be separated in order to understand the illness and possible psychological needs.

I knew after the first diagnosis that I would have to take charge of my healing, because there was no hope offered by doctors or other health-caregivers. This is when I embarked on doing my own research, reading and finding the tools to achieve a healthy balance in my life – focusing on mind, body and spirit. I sought out alternative medicine and the tools for healing and well being. I do believe the body can heal itself if we focus on inner healing of mind and spirit.

I am dealing with change and the stress that comes with it. The stress of continuing on with Nutri-Metics. Still feel a lot of "shoulds" on my part but I know I need to let go of it ALL and focus on healing.

Stress of health and well being – trying to keep up with all the relaxation, visualization, physio, nutrition, bible and other readings, plus prayer. It seems like I'm spending too much time on self and can't see or feel improvements in my physical condition. I feel things happening in my right hand, not unlike the weaknesses that took place in my left hand one year ago, (i.e. in writing and other fine tuning activities). Also my speech – my tongue seems to be lazy. Am I back to the first diagnosis? I need to write an action plan on what I can control and what I can't do – let go.

We sold our home on 23 Scenic Glen Close in the first twelve hours it was listed on the 24th of March. Another stressful situation. The thought of leaving this beautiful home. We did so much work here and built so many beautiful memories. But I guess we can always build more. I'm so thankful for my family. They are all so gentle, loving and sensitive and all have such a great sense of humor. Thank you God for this blessing of loving family and extended family and Mom.

Had a great Easter dinner at Sandy and Denny's with boys and extended family. Also farewell to Mom as she'll be leaving for Provost in a week. More houses to look at. There is always a compromise of a yard, or kitchen, or closets, or lots of repairs.

It is now February, 1999 and I am concluding this chapter. As ALS invades more of my body, each new handicap presents more challenges and frustrations. It is like climbing Mount Everest. I keep my focus on the top, one step at a time. I do not look below or back at what might have been and I pray for God's strength to deal with each new day.

The challenges from the neck up are numerous. My breathing is very shallow and loud, which interferes with my ability to hear the television and listen to music. My eyes blink involuntarily sometimes, which confuses people who mistakenly think I am responding yes to a question. When I am in distress, I cannot blink at all. It seems as though all my muscles tense up when I'm stressed or cold. My facial muscles and tongue are paralyzed, which makes it difficult to drink as much as one sip of water from a glass. I cannot even move a tiny piece of food to the back of my mouth to swallow it.

When my teeth are brushed, I cannot keep my mouth open without clamping down on the toothbrush several times. Saliva drools constantly because I can't swallow very often and someone is constantly wiping my mouth. At the end of the day my mouth and lips burn from the bleach in the Kleenex. Often I eat Kleenex pieces and get teased for wanting it folded into two-inch squares whenever I get transferred. There is a good reason for this. If it is bunched up, pieces stick to my tongue or lips.

Many functions are affected when facial muscles are paralyzed. I cannot have a full sneeze and when yawning, my front teeth bite down on my bottom lip. Larry and I often talk about how much we miss each other's kisses. My nieces and nephews would refer to me as the smooch monster. I love children and would kiss them from their nose to their toes. You can imagine how disheartening it is to be unable to kiss our two grandchildren.

I do not have the energy to cough or blow my nose and caregivers twirl tissue up my nose to clean it. Sometimes my head will drop down very hard because of weakening neck muscles.

The challenges and discomforts from the neck down are also numerous. At the time of this writing, I can still stand with assistance while being transferred and I'm determined to give it my best shot. It is my only act of independence. I marvel now at how God created the human body with so many functions and talents.

I have very little balance, and if my feet, arms or hands are not positioned properly on the wheelchair, recliner, or toilet, I topple to one side. At times, bed can be a torture chamber. I am very grateful for the wonderful care I receive every day and night. I know that I would not receive this quality care in a hospital or hospice.

The things I miss the most are outings, long conversations and reading. Bedtime is now 8:00 or 9:00 P.M. due to fatigue and waking up so many times throughout the night. My body doesn't care, but my mind and heart want to be in the living room with family and friends. How I miss those long conversations that I so enjoyed.

I have cabin fever and the only change of view I get is when my recliner is turned around. My last outing was in November '98. I miss dinner parties and the great outdoors and wish now that I would have taken my son Jarret up on his offer to take me to see the mountain meadows.

I hope heaven has a very large library, but it probably isn't necessary. I prefer reading to watching television, but now that isn't possible. Family and friends read to me, which I enjoy very much.

The biggest barrier between me and the people around me is my inability to communicate, which creates so many misunderstandings. I have listened in dismay to how family or caregivers would interpret why they or I got frustrated or upset. Often their interpretation is far from the truth.

There are incidents like being seated too far to one side of the wheelchair, which causes my head to drop to one side. This twists my spine, causing my feet to go forward on the footrest of the wheelchair. The pain is like a knife in my back and, because I can't call out, I react with tears.

My husband thinks I am having a snit fit, so he sits down to wait until I get over it. In the meantime I am in a great deal of pain and I look at him with eyes of desperation, which he interprets as a look of anger. My shoulders and head are hanging over to one side and I wonder why he can't see that I am not seated properly. He is either distracted in thought or he has forgotten that I need to be centered in the wheelchair. There are so many similar situations that occur in bed, in the recliner or on the toilet.

At the point when my neck became so weak that my head would drop with a thud, I asked my son Jarret to put signs up in the bathroom to remind people to lift my head up whenever it drops. It took the family and caregivers three months before it would be done consistently. When my head drops, it feels like a fifty-pound weight, hanging off a neck that is no longer supported because the muscle has wasted away. This puts stress on the spine and is very painful.

Often people ask me questions while my head is down. Questions about which parts of my body need to be adjusted. How can I begin to answer them? I can only communicate with my eyes and that is impossible when my head is down. I react with tears. Why can they not see what is happening? And then they ask me why I'm crying.

I am now unable to swallow much saliva and I choke if my head is held back. When this happens I go into distress, because the saliva pools in the back of my mouth, choking me. In bed I will choke if my pillow is not propped up correctly.

There are the times when there is a hair on my face and they cannot see it. Again, I wonder why. They ask "What is the matter"? After exhausting me with questions, I look toward the board to spell it out.

When I am on the toilet, caregivers will be concerned about my head dropping down, so they will hold my head up and ask me questions to which I cannot nod "no", I can merely blink "yes". This creates confusion and I can only respond with tears of frustration, wondering why they cannot see that I am unable to respond when they are holding my head.

Pages could be written about misunderstandings, but I don't want to create the impression that I'm ungrateful. I know it's frustrating for caregivers as well, when they don't understand what it is I'm trying to communicate.

Of all the adjustments I have had to make, and all the losses I've had to accept concerning ALS, the inability to communicate has certainly been the most difficult.

The following poem is my own composition to which my friend Rachael Owens composed the music at my request. The song will appear on a CD, which will be recorded soon, and she will donate one dollar to the ALS Society for every CD sold. The song is entitled ALS.

A L S

ALS can take away all my physical abilities,
walking, talking and writing,
But it can't take away my spirit.
It leaves my mind and senses, for that I am grateful.
It can't take away my sense of humor.
It can't take away my faith, hope or love.
It can't take away the many treasured memories,
Or the wisdom gained from life's experiences.
It can't take away my relationship with God, or family or friends.
It can put a dent in my dignity, but I have plenty.
It can't take away the joy and laughter in our home.
It can instill fear about the journey, but not the destination;
But with God walking alongside of me, I will triumph over ALS.

Evelyn Bell

CHAPTER SIX

Family & Friends - A Year in Review

January, 1998

The workload at school and at home was taking its toll on Larry, so he took a three-month leave of absence from school. We decided to go to Phoenix, Arizona. With Larry holding me upright under my arms, I was still able to walk and get into a plane seat from a wheelchair. I did not drink anything on the plane because I could not walk to the bathroom. The seat was very uncomfortable but I endured. My mother came with us to help, as well as to enjoy the sights and sounds of Phoenix. We stayed three weeks in a lovely condo and the weather was perfect for me. With ALS, if it is too hot, you wilt and get very weak. If it is too cold, your muscles tense up and teeth chatter. The desert was very beautiful with its array of succulent plants.

We would take walks every morning along the streets lined with orange and grapefruit trees that were bending with the weight of the fruit. What a waste to see so much fruit on the ground. Larry's parents came from Yuma to see us while we were there and we visited some relatives and friends as well. I now recall the wide variety of foods that I could still eat, compared to the four foods that I am limited to now. On our return, we had a twelve-hour delay because of plane repairs. It was impossible for me to stay at the airport. We woke up our good friend, Sally Stotts, and retired to her place for most of that time. We were all exhausted when we returned home.

On the days that followed, I reflected on our holiday and how much different it would have been if I had been healthy. Dancing, hiking and trying different restaurants would have been our thing to do. But we cannot focus on what could have been. I was always a very active person and can't help but think creatively about what I want to do next.

February, 1998

After contacting an agency, we found a caregiver, Tina Braun, who worked two hours a day, in the mornings. She is still with us. She is very compassionate and dedicated and always finds something to clean when she is not caring for me.

My mother assists with certain routines and makes our home permeate with the wonderful aroma of her baking and the delicious meals she prepares daily. I often wonder how many mothers would give up their home and lifestyle to care for one of their adult children. It would be a huge workload for Larry if he had to prepare meals and do laundry and other household chores. We are truly blessed to have a mother who is so loving, giving and generous with her time.

Larry looks after me when the caregiver leaves, usually from 5:00 P.M. until I go to bed. My husband is very dedicated and lovingly cares for me. We have been through some tough times in our thirty-one years together but we have always triumphed. God is testing us in what will surely be the test of our lives.

Our sons help out whenever their schedules allow. They are eager to help and they do so lovingly. Christy, our daughter-in-law, prepares meals when she visits, which gives my mom a break.

February was the month that marked the end of walking, which was from the sink to the toilet. I persisted until my feet were too heavy to lift. It was hard to accept yet another freedom taken by ALS. I surprised myself that I did not go into a state of panic or depression. The gradual loss of my ability to walk gave me time to accept the inevitable. It was only six months from the time I needed assistance to walk, which was August of '97, to February '98, when I could no longer walk at all. That was all the time it took for ALS to cast its destruction.

March, 1998

Family and friends, some uncles, aunts and cousins come to visit. These visits are usually greeted and ended with tears of joy mainly because a person with ALS does not have the muscle control to hold back the tears. I have to tell people that, so they don't think they have upset me. Visits always provide the support I need from time to time.

Some friends and relatives do not visit at all, and that hurts. My friend, Mert Trent told me about her response to someone who told her that she could not handle my disease. Mert replied "You aren't dealing with ALS, Evelyn is!" That shows that people see the disease and not me. I have not changed. I am still the same person. One of the reasons I am writing this book is to create awareness and understanding about the disease. During visits, people will rarely ask me questions about the disease, but instead, will request written information.

Cards, letters, faxes and bouquets of flowers arrive weekly from family, friends and relatives. I am extremely grateful for this support. I delight when I hear the fax machine working or when Larry brings the mail, because this is my link to the outside world.

I so enjoyed the book "Waiting for a Miracle" by Jan Markell, that I ordered twelve copies to give to family and friends. Although it took a long time, I wrote a -special message in each book. My son Jarret's birthday is in March, so I wrote a birthday letter for all three sons because I knew it would be my last writing. My right hand was becoming more difficult to move and by the end of March, I surrendered my last limb to ALS.

April, 1998

It is now two years since I first experienced the clumsiness in my left hand. I can't believe how fast ALS has taken over my body. It is relentless and I am still trying to get used to the paralysis and being so totally dependent on other people. Sometimes I feel a strong urge to jump out of my wheelchair and run. Sometimes I want to scream! Scream at the top of my lungs – enough already!

Quality of life is very limited when you spend it in three places – the wheelchair, recliner and bed. I think of the many diseases and accidents that cause people to become housebound and I realize the pain we have in common, emotional pain, and for some, much physical pain.

The organizers of the annual Betty Run notified me that I had been chosen as this year's ambassador. I cried and felt very honored. I was active in the first Betty Run in 1997. Betty and I met at a seminar that we both attended shortly after our diagnoses. Betty was diagnosed in August of '96 and died in July of '97. ALS affects everyone differently and she had the aggressive type.

With Larry's help, I began to make a list of names to mail out brochures. I knew that I would have the support of family and friends and I decided that I would also mail brochures to my former clients in Nutri-Metics because many had also become my friends. The president of Nutri-Metics was kind enough to send brochures to all my colleagues across the country. I was confident that it would be a big success. I then suggested to my sister, Laura, in Lloydminster to hold a run in her city and she responded with great enthusiasm. My mind was full of promotional ideas. If only I could get out of this wheelchair.

May, 1998

Larry and I decided to attend the ALS clinic and I was encouraged to have a feeding tube, called the peg, inserted into my stomach. They told me there was a window of opportunity for inserting the peg and if I delayed, I would miss it. I had mixed feelings about that and I questioned three ALS patients who had the peg. I reasoned that I was eating three meals, each consisting of 1,000 to 1,200 calories daily, which I thought was good for an inactive person, but I had to admit that dehydration was a problem. Drinking liquids was very difficult and the bib got more liquid than I did. Larry always referred to giving me a drink as a test of endurance. After meeting with the specialist who would perform the twenty-minute surgery, I decided that I would go ahead with it. A date was set for July 24th.

The 24th of May was a special day. It saw the birth of our first grandchild, Isaiah. He was born in Nelson, B.C.. Our son Derek sent us a video of his family, which helped us feel as though we were there with them. Derek and Christy said they would come for a visit in three or four weeks and we looked forward to that visit with great anticipation.

June, 1998

My sister, Laura and her husband Peter organized a very successful run for ALS in Lloydminster, which raised $7,000.00. What awareness could be raised if people in more towns and cities would organize a simple fundraiser so it could become a national event annually.

The second annual Betty Run was held on a bright, sunny day. When my family and I arrived, there was already a large crowd of people waiting. The sight of so many familiar faces was overwhelming. Everyone took their turn to greet us with affection and eagerness.

The other ambassador for the event was Mark Baird. When I saw him arrive, I broke down and cried. His disease was more advanced than mine and I couldn't help but feel all his pain. His daughter is a student at Sir Winston Churchill High School where my husband is a guidance counsellor. Larry had spoken several times about ALS during student assemblies, which created the support of many students who participated in the run.

There were four hundred people that either walked or ran that day and $85,000 was raised. From that amount, approximately $15,000 came from our family and friends. We were overwhelmed with this support and ever so grateful.

The following speech was written by Evelyn and delivered by Larry at the "Betty Run".

A year ago I was walking and standing on my own here at the Betty Run. Today I am wheelchair bound and totally dependent on the four men in my life, my husband, Larry, our sons Derek, Jarret and Travis. Also my daughter-in-law, Christy, my mother Betty and caregivers Tina and Bruce. Life has changed dramatically for our family.

Betty Norman was diagnosed in August and I was diagnosed in November of 1996. I remember meeting Betty at a seminar that fall and we discussed our concerns. I will never forget the look in her eyes as we said goodbye. That look spoke volumes of the feelings one has to deal with when afflicted with ALS. Amongst the feelings of isolation, desperation and dependency is the disbelief that there is still not a cure or known cause for this mysterious disease. Did you know that more people die of ALS than AIDS? The majority of people do not know what ALS is, yet how many people in the world know about AIDS? The most shocking news, besides being diagnosed with ALS, was the fact that there wasn't a cure or a known cause for it. ALS is a very cruel disease. It takes away all your physical freedoms. It is unrelenting and your body slowly becomes a wasteland of paralyzed muscles. Your intellect and senses stay intact and trapped in a dying body. I feel like I am living on an island watching the world go by. The most difficult part is not being able to communicate spontaneously and to hug and kiss my loved ones, especially a new grandson. Thank goodness for a spelling board and laser light and three new friends, Shawna Kinniburg, Janie Walton and Bernice Clark, who each scribe for me one morning a week in my home. I can still turn my head from side to side and stand up briefly while someone is holding me. Also, I can swallow, but not chew. I will be getting a feeding tube shortly. The fatigue is constant with ALS.

Emotionally, there are a lot of feelings to sort through and every day is a challenge. I deal with it by trusting in God's care and taking one day at a time. Spiritually, I focus on the eternal goal, which keeps my spirits and hopes high.

Today I would like to acknowledge all those afflicted with ALS and encourage each of you to rely on God's strength. He is walking with us in this journey. So hang in there!

I would like to acknowledge my family, my sisters, brothers and their families. Also our cousins and many friends who are supporting this cause. Thank you, I appreciate all of you. I also want to thank those who could no be here, but made a donation. Donations came in from as far away as Indonesia, Toronto, Vancouver and Victoria. My sister Laura held a run, which raised $7,100. Thank you to all the participants here today for helping create awareness and finding a cure for ALS. Hopefully, people will now have the courage to talk and ask questions about ALS with those afflicted with ALS.

I appreciate all those who have given so much of their time to this cause. I would like to show my appreciation to Jane Rivest of the ALS Society and Kelly Eaton, daughter of Betty Norman, who helped organize this event to make it a success. Individually and collectively, everyone here today has made a difference.

My family and I are grateful to "Betty and Friends" and to all of you here today. Thank you. We appreciate you. Hope to see you next year.

July, 98

My neck was getting weaker to the point where I needed a neck support on my wheelchair so that my head would not drop forward so often. My head feels like a fifty-pound weight and sometimes takes more energy than I have just to lift it. When I eat or drink, my head goes down for easier swallowing.

My relatives, Sally and Gerry Stotts organized a golf tournament and dinner in my honor at Pinebrook Golf and Country Club, to raise awareness and funding for ALS. Again I felt very honored and grateful for the opportunity to help people become more aware. We sent a mailing list to Sally, who did all the organizing for the event. I assured Sally that I would be there with bells on, even though I was to have the stomach tube surgery two days prior to the event.

The tubes that were inserted down my throat into my stomach were extremely unpleasant and caused a lot of discomfort. It seemed like an eternity while the tubes were going up and down and in and out. I stayed one night in the hospital and Larry stayed with me. Thank God he did, because nurses were scarce and did not understand what I was communicating with only my eyes. Bruce, my caregiver was with me in the afternoon and I was so grateful that he was there to communicate for me. It would have been a nightmare without him because they wanted to flip me on to my stomach for X-rays and he told them that they could not do that because I had just had a stomach tube inserted. I would die if I had to go through that surgery again, but was glad that I had it done, and relieved that it was over.

Two days later, my family and I attended the golf and dinner fundraiser. It was a very warm evening with a magnificent sunset. Many friends were there, including those that we hadn't seen for a few years. Some relatives made the trip from Milk River, Lethbridge and Pincher Creek. We were elated with the turnout. The dinner was a feast for the eyes and although I could not eat anything, I enjoyed watching others eat. There were many gifts donated and most people went home with a prize. The silent auction was very successful. At the close of the evening, many came to offer me great encouragement and some told me about losing their spouse to ALS. It was Gerry Stotts' speech about how much the government designated last year to ALS that spurred me to write a book. People were shocked to hear that it was only $15,000. I'd assumed that it would have been in the millions. After all, it is a 130 year-old disease with still no known cause or cure. Wouldn't that deserve some serious attention? The golf and dinner raised $11,000 for ALS.

The following is a letter of gratitude written by Evelyn and delivered by Larry.

My family and I would like to thank everyone for participating in this event to help raise awareness for ALS. We are deeply grateful to Gerry and Sally Stotts for all their efforts in planning and organizing this event. We know the many phone calls Sally had to make to keep this thing moving. Your generosity of time and resources has no boundaries. We appreciate you so much.

I thought it would help if I communicated with you by letter, since I cannot speak. Some of you have asked if I have feeling in my limbs, which I do. Some think I am deaf, because they speak louder. Well, I am not deaf. And still others question my mind. Well, don't feel bad. My family and I didn't know about ALS and how it affects the body either. I thought I would share a little about ALS with you to create greater awareness about this mysterious disease. ALS is a disease that is over 130 years old. More people die from ALS than AIDS! Everyone knows about AIDS but too few know about ALS. The most shocking and devastating news for me was that there is no cure because they do not know what causes it. It is better known as Lou Gehrig's disease – named after the baseball player. Seven out of a hundred thousand get ALS. Usually it hits more men, and later in life. The life expectancy is two to five years.

ALS attacks motor neurons, which are among the largest of all the nerve cells in the brain and spinal cord. These cells send messages to muscles throughout the body. In ALS, motor neurons die and the muscles do not receive these messages. As a result, the muscles weaken as they lose their ability to move. Eventually, most muscle action is affected, including those which control swallowing and breathing, as well as major muscles in the arms, legs, back and neck.

There is, however, no loss of sensory nerves, so people with ALS retain their sense of feeling, sight, hearing, smell and taste. This disease does not affect the mind and people with ALS remain fully alert and aware of events.

One year ago, I was driving, talking, walking, and had use of my right hand. I still wake up some mornings and think I am just having a bad dream. When you look at me, you may think I haven't physically changed aside from the muscle and weight loss. My body is a wasteland of paralyzed muscles, but my mind is alert and filled with creative energy, trapped in a dying body.

Today I can only stand for a few minutes. I spend my time between the wheelchair, recliner and the bed. I communicate with a spelling board and a laser light and the help of friends. I watch a little television, read the Bible, and other books, when I have someone to turn the pages. I can't chew food, but I can swallow when food is pureed. The fatigue is constant with ALS.

People ask how I deal with this affliction. I live out my dying, one day at a time. I have complete faith and confidence in our Lord. I trust that He is walking this journey with me and I have nothing to fear. I try everyday to focus on the eternal goal rather than the things of the world. I give thanks for the people in my life and all the blessings, which keep my perspective on life.

I am blessed with a loving family that saturates me with love each day. Also a loving mother and husband who look after so many of my needs. I am grateful for the many people and caregivers who help with my physical and emotional needs.

I would like to thank all those who helped to make this event successful. I would also like to show our gratitude to the sponsors of the prizes. And again, our deepest gratitude to you, Sally and Gerry, for giving of yourselves. You are so special. Thank you everyone for attending. Individually and collectively, everyone here today has made a difference in finding a cure for ALS. Thank you.

August/98

The tube feed was going well and I was glad that I'd had it done. I would recommend it to other ALS patients. People who came to visit commented that I now had some color and weight on my face. Now I can eat for pleasure without being concerned about nutrition.

My diet is limited to pureed food, pudding, ice cream and anything that is easy to swallow because I can't chew or roll the food in my mouth with a paralyzed tongue. How I would love to bite into a Caesar salad or a sandwich. I don't get hungry on the tube feed but I do crave foods that I can't eat.

Our youngest son, Travis has been home working since March and had to make a tough decision about where to play hockey. He could go back to B.C. for his final year or go to U of C to play for the Dinos. He felt that he should be home because of my illness, but he was also torn because he wanted to play out his last season of junior hockey. I told him that whatever he decided, I would support him. I could tell it was weighing heavy on his mind. His coach reassured him that he could fly home once a month to visit so he made the decision to go back to Duncan to play for the Cowichan Valley Capitals of the B.C. hockey league. It was hard to see him go, but I knew it would be only one month before he would be home again.

September/98

In September we had an unusual amount of visitors. We travelled to Edmonton to visit my sister Vel and her family and it was nice to get out and about. I tolerated the trip quite well except for the turns in the road, which rocked me from side to side.

My spine is getting weaker and I can't adjust my upper body. Travis and my mom would say, "Don't let yourself fall over in the chair". They didn't realize that I was getting weaker and that I could not adjust myself or hold myself up.

I have now written three chapters of my book and feel very good about that. I am very grateful for my friends and niece who scribe for me, to help me finish this book.

My dear friend, Judy Howard arranged for CFCN Television to do a feature story on the book and me. I was grateful for the opportunity to raise awareness about ALS and was hoping to get the attention of some government officials.

Jarret returned to the U of C for his last term, and will graduate in the spring of '99. He makes time for family visits and dinner every week and massages my hands and feet or he will read to me.

October/98

Larry asked if I realized that if I did not have the tube I would be dead by now. I did realize that and was grateful that I'd made the decision to have it, because it added quality to my life. The amount of food that I was eating amounted to about 200 calories a day. When I eat, I get exhausted from holding my head up and my breathing is very labored.

Travis came home for a four-day visit and at the same time, Derek, Christy, Jasmine and baby Isaiah arrived as well. They said they had a surprise for me. Sunday evening dinner was hurried and Christy asked if she could gather up all the candles in the house and place them in the living room. They moved my chair and other furniture around. At 7:00 P.M. the doorbell rang and four people dressed in tuxedos, carrying musical instruments, walked in and proceeded to set up their four string quartet under the chandelier.

When they played their first piece I was overwhelmed and could not hold back the tears. They played all my favorites from Bach and other classical compositions. It was like having a concert in my own home. What a great gift from Derek and Christy and some of their friends in Edgewood. An outing to see a concert is impossible for me, but this was perfect because I could enjoy it with my family. I will always treasure the memory.

November/98

It is two years on November 7th, 1998 since my first diagnosis of ALS. It is a relentless disease, and in two years is has captured my mobility, speech and now the joy of eating. It became such a struggle to swallow the five spoonfuls I was eating for breakfast and dinner, I gave up. So now the only taste in my mouth is that of toothpaste every morning and evening. My breathing has become labored and when the room is too warm I find it difficult to breathe. The nights are sometimes a torture test because of the pressure and gurgling mucus. My protruding tailbone has no padding and throbs with pain all night long. I communicated this to my family doctor and he recommended liquid morphine that could be syringed into my stomach tube. I had already tried an anti-inflammatory that made me constipated for a week, so I gave morphine a chance. I did not sleep better, nor did it take the pain away completely, but it kept me drowsy for the two days I was on it. It also caused constipation for over a week, which was so uncomfortable I decided no more morphine. My caregivers put Nutri-Rich Oil on my tailbone and back five times a day, which helped to minimize the pressure points.

November 11th was our 31st wedding anniversary. We decided to celebrate it by having the Wild Rose String Quartet come once again to our house to play. I wanted to celebrate it with my family and the six volunteers that come to scribe for me and Larry thought it was a good idea. It was a very memorable evening with our own concert and great company. I drew a lot of energy from the music and fine guests.

My sisters, Laura and Vel came to help Larry and mom for the weekend. Vel decorated our home for Christmas, while Laura and Peter grocery shopped and prepared meals. I am so very grateful to them. They come almost every month to provide whatever help is needed. Our very good friends Adeline and her daughter Shannon came to help on another weekend.

My husband Larry is my main caregiver. In the past year he has given up all of his social life to look after me. I am so blessed and grateful for his dedication and loving care. We have our challenging moments, but we always forgive and forget. He is with me every evening. Sometimes he doesn't get very much sleep and it's hard on him when he has to go to work the next morning. We no longer go out for visits or dinner dates since I have become weaker. It is difficult to find the words to express what my heart feels for him. I will be eternally grateful for his devoted love and care of me in the more challenging times that we will be soon facing.

I wonder how many mothers would give up their lifestyle to take care of family needs. Our family is so very appreciative of her. I am grateful for her care when Larry or caregivers are not present. She is a special mother with a very big heart.

Our three sons and daughter-in-law help whenever they are home. They are quick to help with transfers, give me hand and foot massages, brush my teeth or do whatever needs to be done. I feel so good in their arms because it is like a hug from them. Although they give me lots of kisses and hugs, I cannot reciprocate, which is very frustrating. I can see the love in their eyes and we wink at each other to say, "I love you". My sisters and sister-in-law also help on a regular basis, for which Larry and I are very grateful.

December, 1998

I woke up this December morning reflecting on the happenings of 1998. I get so annoyed with myself at night because my mind is alert when it should be comatose. I recall where I was healthwise last December and where I am now, a year later. ALS has held me captive and imprisoned me in this lifeless body.

I think about the many tears I've shed in the last two years, which I can honestly say were more than in all the other combined years of my life. There are tears of sadness, tears of joy, tears of frustration, tears of helplessness and desperation, tears of anxiety and tears of being loved so much.

It is still a constant challenge to master my thoughts and control my emotions. Anxiety and fatigue are my constant companions because I am so totally dependent on others. Even though I place my trust in family and caregivers, I have no control when they are not focused or forget to position me properly.

If you could measure emotional or spiritual progress, I would say I have come a distance since the beginning of the year.

Physically I have deteriorated and it is certain that I would have starved to death had it not been for the feeding tube. I missed all the Christmas meals and chocolates since I no longer eat or drink anything orally. I can still enjoy the aroma of my mom's baking and cooking as it wafts through our house.

It has been six weeks with our new caregiver, Janice Richard, and both Larry and I are very pleased with her. She is only 25 years old and catches on quickly to not only the routine, but also to my short vocabulary and eye expressions. She is consistent in her routine, which reduces frustration and I feel very calm and relaxed in her care. I am grateful for the caregivers we have.

Travis had his twentieth birthday on December 2, the same day that he had to fly to Cornell in New York state. He was very impressed with the Ivy League University and the caliber of hockey. This would be a four-year hockey scholarship and it was a gutwrenching decision for him. Should he stay because his mom was dying? He could play for the Dinosaurs while attending the University of Calgary. This would please his father because he could finally watch his son play hockey.

Travis enlisted the family to help make the big decision. I told him I would not want to stand in his way. I asked him what his goal was and encouraged him to follow his dream while I assured him that his dad and I would support him in whatever decision he made. He had until the end of December to decide and, with the family's support, he made the four-year commitment to Cornell.

Christmas was a wonderful celebration with just the immediate family. Derek made the Christmas dinner, which consisted of salmon, shrimp and several side dishes that smelled divine. I sat with the family and looked on as everyone devoured their meal. I could remember how every bit of that food tasted. At 1: 00 P.M. we had mass celebrated in our home, which was very special, thanks to Mark and Father John, our priest.

This Christmas was special because of baby Isaiah. He was seven months old and celebrating his first Christmas. It was such a joy to hear his happy sounds everyday during his one-week visit with us.

All the excitement caused me to become extremely exhausted and I did not sleep well. ALS is capturing more of the mobility in my neck, which causes my head to fall hard. When that happens, it takes all the energy I can muster to lift it up. Instead of getting one page done for my book, I am now completing two or three paragraphs. Volunteers have to lift my head and continually wipe my mouth while processing the words.

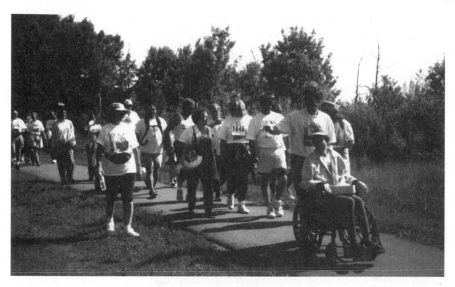

Betty's Run for ALS, June 1998

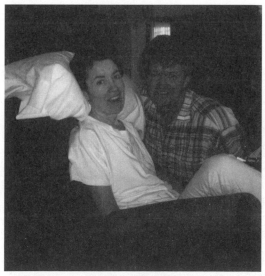

Evelyn & Larry

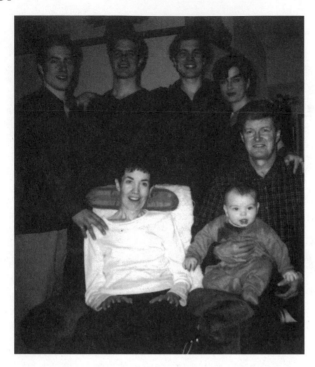

Evelyn with Travis, Jarret, Derek, Christy, Larry and Isaiah

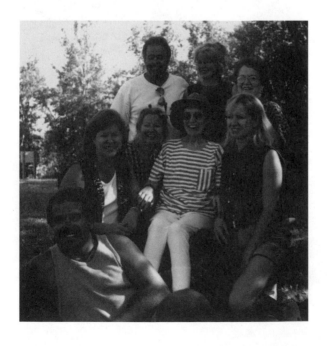

Evelyn with her siblings Kon, Vel, Mother Betty, Laura, Joanne, Sandy and James

CHAPTER SEVEN

Bringing ALS
out of the Dark Ages

Many studies have been done to determine the cause of ALS. Recent research has led to promising new clues that are being examined. Some of the areas of particular interest are environmental factors such as exposure to heavy metals, dietary deficiencies, viruses and massive overdoses of insecticide. As yet, no one knows the cause, but they do know that it is not contagious or anything a patient can knowingly do to oneself. No one can "catch" ALS.

At the time of my three diagnoses, I questioned why I wasn't asked about environmental and nutritional factors. The only questions I was asked had to do with family history. There is a belief held by some doctors and dentists that amalgam fillings leak mercury into our systems, which may cause neurological damage. What is one to believe when there is such controversy about ALS?

I do not have answers, only a lot of questions. If it is true that breast cancer and heart disease can be reduced with a nutritious diet, wouldn't it also be reasonable to think that proper nutrition could play a part in the cure of other diseases? Doctors admit that in their medical training, nutrition plays a very small part.

Then there is the subject of treatments through alternative medicine. Some of these include vitamins, herbs and acupuncture. This too is controversial. Why is the scientific community not spending more time researching preventative medicine?

Eastern medicines have helped cure many diseases. I feel that we could learn and benefit from it. Wouldn't it be a step in the right direction if eastern and traditional medicine and treatment were available under one roof? Could they not complement each other? It is difficult, when I don't have the use of my hands and feet, which would allow me to provide factual information regarding what I have written so far in this chapter. I can only tell you what my experience has been.

At the onset of my diagnosis, I read many books pertaining to health and wellness and tried many different things that I thought would benefit me. Some were very costly, some worked, and some didn't. There was the feeling of frustration and being exploited at a time when I was extremely vulnerable. During my experimental phase, I questioned why there could not be a body, mind and soul clinic for the terminally and chronically ill. I thought about the many patients I would see with bitter faces, when I would go to the hospital. I wondered how many would at some point give up and throw in the towel. Some of them do not have any family support. I could see the misery on their faces.

I do believe that if doctors do not treat the whole person, body, mind and soul, there is less chance for healing to take place. Some patients do not have faith or the coping skills to heal themselves, but a clinic of this nature could provide the tools and direction for them to start the healing process. They may not be physically healed, but emotionally and spiritually they could heal themselves and find peace and well-being within. How strange that man has conquered outer space but remains so far from conquering inner space.

The human body is very complex. The physical, emotional and spiritual lives are intertwined. Modern medical practitioners must become more aware of how they address and deal with these issues to empower the afflicted. If our own emotional and spiritual lives are in balance, we can make a difference in people's lives.

CHAPTER EIGHT

Public & Government Awareness

Every person that knows about ALS can make a difference by becoming involved in fundraisers. Those that are afflicted with ALS are too fatigued and some, like me, are mute and unable to speak out about this relentless disease. We can however, make appearances at events so people can have an idea of how ALS affects the body and not the mind.

We can also influence our family and friends to get involved and help create awareness for research in finding the cause and cure. Another way that ALS patients can create awareness is by being interviewed for television, radio or newspaper coverage. It does take courage for us to be exposed in a vulnerable state. Sometimes a visual makes more impact than words.

There are many corporations that would make annual donations if they were aware of the need for ALS research and equipment. This is where you, the reader can get involved. I would like to encourage corporations to sponsor fundraisers like the Betty Run and the Pinebrook Golf Tournament, which are both annual events. The question comes to mind whether corporations would consider sponsoring airtime for ALS awareness. Billboards would also help.

Equipment and technical devices are needed for daily use by ALS patients but the way things are now, one has to wait for wheelchairs, mattresses and other essentials to become available through Daily Aids for Living.

Technical devices like my laser light should be plentiful, so that when it breaks down, another one is available. It is my lifeline. It is the only way I can communicate.

I was given a letter board with the laser and I, with the help of my family, created my own wordboard, with includes the most commonly used words. In addition to this, I also added messages of my needs, and words of appreciation. A word/letter board and laser light could be made more accessible to ALS patients.

I've tried a suction machine but it is very inconvenient, because when it is needed, caregivers have to turn it on end, and by then it is too late to catch the mucus. It is too big and noisy to sit on my lap for easy access. Somewhere there has to be a hand held suction gadget that is as accessible as a tissue. The suction part that goes in the mouth and throat is not as good a fit as the equipment used by dentists. Then the question comes to mind, who designs these suctions machines, and do they get feedback from ALS patients?

It has been our experience with homecare agencies that when a caregiver was unable to come, they would send a substitute who was a total stranger to us, and who had never worked with ALS patients before. This is unfair to both the caregiver and the patient. How could they expect that person to communicate with someone who is mute, especially when they don't know the routine?

This is just one example of the many oversights that occurred with the first agency we used. There is no specialized training for caregivers that work with ALS patients. I would ask them about their training and what experience they had with ALS but the answer was always "none". I would like to see an agency that primarily deals with ALS, who could offer specialized training, which would reduce anxiety, frustration and fatigue.

When caregivers were sent, it was obvious from their actions, questions and comments that they were not aware of ALS or how it affects the body. Even the family that is with me more than caregivers does not fully understand what is happening when the disease is progressing. I spell it out for them when we get frustrated and leave feedback for caregivers and family.

I cannot use the laser light in bed because I cannot turn my head from side to side when it is sunk into the pillow. The discomfort, anxiety and frustration are described very accurately in the following article that my dear friend Judy Howard wrote on my behalf.

It is my sincere desire that you will do more than merely read the words on this page. I ask that you will, for a few minutes, journey into the world of ALS. This is the only way to truly grasp the devastation of this horrifying relentless disease.

Imagine waking up in the middle of the night, either for no apparent reason, or perhaps nudged by your bladder, as we all do from time to time. Now visualize that you have ALS. Your mind is vibrant and very much alive, but your body has become a living corpse. You are unable to move one muscle. You want to turn to a more comfortable position, but you can't. You are totally and completely paralyzed. But what you still have is all the feeling and sensation you always had. The difference is that now you are hypersensitive. All of your senses have become more acute. You lie there becoming more and more uncomfortable. You feel pressure points on your hip and your arm is tingling due to lack of circulation from lying in one position too long, but there is nothing you can do about it. Now you are feeling an itch somewhere on your body, you can't scratch, so you lie there, hoping it will go away. But now another itch has developed and you feel as though there are insects crawling on you. The agitation begins. You are helpless. There is absolutely nothing you can do for yourself. You must lie there, wondering if your mind is strong enough to tolerate this and keep your sanity. You have reached a point where you want to scream.

Now you know you can't endure it for one second longer. You must call out to someone, anyone, who can come and move you. But you can't call out. ALS has paralyzed your tongue. You can no longer speak. You can only utter sounds to awaken your spouse, nurse or caregiver out of a dead sleep. They come to your bed wondering what is wrong with you, but you cannot tell them. Now they must go through a series of questions to try to determine what it is that is bothering you, but you cannot articulate. You can only shake your head to communicate the answer no and blink for yes. They must ask the right question, and sometimes that can take forever. On a good night you will awaken your caregiver four times, on a bad night, a dozen times.

Perhaps you have to use the toilet. You cannot hop out of bed like you used to. The caregiver must lift your lifeless body out of the bed, put you in the wheelchair, lift you onto the toilet and then do the same in reverse to put you back to bed. Now they must go through the procedure of positioning your body, limb by limb into just the right position for you to be able to sleep. The pillow must be perfect to alleviate pain in the neck or back. The blankets must be perfect and the weight not too heavy on your body. Your night-clothes must be free of any wrinkles or they will dig into you. This whole procedure can take up to an hour, because comfort is imperative to be able to sleep.

You eventually do fall asleep, but you awaken an hour later. You are cold. The lack of circulation in your body has turned your hands and feet to what feel like ice cubes. Again, there is nothing you can do. You can't merely pull up or add more covers, you must, again, alert your caregiver and attempt to convey what is wrong this time.

Nights can seem to last forever when you have ALS. Days are a whole other story. A story that a person without the disease could not even begin to imagine.

The specialty training that I am referring to would involve the following points for family, caregivers and ALS patients:

1. Language should be positive at all times to create a higher energy level and reduce anxiety and fatigue.

2. Proper transfers will help ALS patients to support their own weight. It has been my experience that all caregivers have the same style of transfer. I have found that if their knees were braced directly in front of mine, it would enable me to snap out of the chair. If they use their own method of squeezing my knees between their knees, I would have less mobility to snap up.

3. Many times, ALS patients are put in a state of discomfort unintentionally. An example would be having a caregiver moving the patient's shoulders without bringing them forward first. When this happens in the chair or bed, it creates wrinkles in my shirt, which causes pressure points, especially on bedsores.

4. As the neck gets weaker, ALS patients cannot turn their head around to point with their eyes at things behind or beside them, like when they want such things as the door open or the heat

adjusted. Family and caregivers tend to stick to routine instead of being more aware of the environment. It would help if they would think with their body and how comfortable they would like their body to be.

5. In addition to being a caregiver that is compassionate and patient, it requires someone who can comprehend directions and internalize them. They should not take feedback personally, but should realize that it is the only way an ALS patient can communicate with laser or computer.

6. I highly recommend that both family and caregivers try the following assignments:

   (a) spend a day in a wheelchair with someone pushing you around. This will create awareness about how patients cannot see what is behind or beside them.

   (b) wear a neck brace or have your head on a headrest so you will become aware of the limitations they create.

   (c) attempt to spend one night lying in one position on your back with your arms beside your body - this will create an awareness of several things.

   (d) have someone transfer you on the toilet, into bed and into a recliner - this will create awareness about the importance of positioning of feet and holding the body upright.

7. Consistency reduces frustration. By this I am referring to being consistent in aligning the body in transfers to wheelchair, recliner and bed.

8. Maintaining focus on what you are doing when with an ALS patient is top priority. If caregivers allow their minds to wonder or engage in conversation, it will risk injuring or putting the patient in a state of discomfort.

9. Family and caregivers need to be more aware of not only the physical, but also the emotional, mental and spiritual needs of the patient. If they cannot be of assistance, they should refer someone who can help. Being cheerful and having a good sense of humor relaxes the patient with ALS. Sarcasm and impatience heightens anxiety and causes muscle tension. When caregivers forget details about their routine, it causes anxiety and increases

frustration for both the patient and the caregiver.

10. It takes a leap of faith for a patient to co-operate fully with their caregiver. It is important to be a good patient, recognizing that quality care takes team effort.

11. Relaxation tapes or meditative music can be helpful for ALS patients, family and caregivers when they are uptight or simply want to reflect.

12. To avoid endless questions, I have found the following to be effective:

    When I am in bed, put questions into three main categories:

    (a) Is it the body?

    (b) Is it something on the body or bed (quilt, sheet, pillow, night clothes, stomach tube?)

    (c) Is it the bed? Which means do I want the head or feet up or down on the adjustable bed, or the vibrator turned on.

    I have a very short vocabulary for the following words that have more than one meaning:

    UP – means one of the following: move my body up in the bed, or head up, or tilt bum up, or it could also mean pull quilt up or sheet up over me and flip me to my side, or turn the pillow over, or move part of my body over so that I am aligned.

    OFF – means take something off, such as pull the quilt or the sheet down, or pull tape off the tube, or take the bum cushion out. I blink when they get it right and I nod for no. If I am too weak to nod, then I just wait for the right answer and then I blink.

    Caregivers have to be alert and remember to ask single and not to ask double questions.

    Do not offer choices. Watch the eyes when you ask questions or need more clarity.

13. ALS patients put their heads down when swallowing food or liquid. Caregivers should not ask questions or talk when a patient is eating or drinking, because it requires concentration. If there is a choking spell, allow the patient to go through it. Do not cover the patient's mouth with tissue. Encourage the patient to breathe through their nose, it is helpful.

14. As swallowing becomes more difficult, it helps to have the patient tilt the head slightly forward to wipe saliva with tissue. I prefer to have caregivers wipe inside my lower lip to absorb excess saliva. If saliva runs down my chin, I will look up to the ceiling as a signal to wipe my chin.

In contrast to other lethal diseases to which the government has allotted millions of dollars, I question why ALS has received so little. Is it due to lack of awareness or is there some other reason? It is a 130-year-old disease. Why hasn't anything significant been done to make an impact on research funding?

It was very shocking to many people, including myself, to discover what the federal government has allotted for ALS research in the past.

However, Health Canada has funded $111,292 for ALS Society of Canada projects in the past six years, and in February 1999, the federal government announced significant new funding for medical research.

The major source of funds for ALS research comes from volunteer work across the country associated with Flower Days and ALS Month in June of each year. The revenue from Flower Day activity is applied immediately to a designated Research Fund. This fund is also built from other donations designated to research. In Alberta, The Betty Run for ALS raises significant dollars every year for research.

A Scientific Advisory Committee, made up of six or seven researchers from various disciplines related to the study of ALS, meets annually to allocate the money available to researchers who have submitted the best and most useful grant proposals. ALS Canada and ALS Societies across Canada are committed to funding only the best research.

The ALS Society of Canada is the only voluntary health organization in Canada dedicated solely to finding a cure for ALS. In 1998, ALS Canada funded $522,813 toward Canadian research projects in the hope of finding a cure for ALS.

ALS is a very cruel disease, which buries an active mind in a paralyzed body with multiple handicaps. Families exhaust their financial resources on supplies and homecare assistance. I propose that the provincial government allocate additional funds to assist families such as mine.

When patients cannot walk, talk, write, eat or sleep and are so totally dependent on others, it would help to lift financial burdens for people with ALS and their families. If an individual were in the hospital it may cost the government far more money than having them cared for at home and the care in an institution is often questionable.

In this province, Alberta Health will provide a power wheelchair to enable an individual to go to work or school. However, they do not provide this equipment for people dealing with chronic, degenerative conditions such as ALS, so that these individuals may go shopping, see their child play ball or perform in a school concert.

They will provide a hospital bed, but again not an electric one, which may be able to be operated by the person with ALS, thereby maintaining some independence and quality of life for much longer.

Family members are often the best care providers. However, funding support from health care does not have any provisions to pay for this assistance. A family member could be in a position to provide help and have to quit gainful employment to assist, but can not receive pay for this assistance.

As an example, a son or daughter may have to quit a good job that pays $30,000 to $40,000 annually and receive nothing to care for a loved one. This does not make much sense and negates the possibility of an excellent care provider from within the family. In fact, no one related to the person requiring care can receive payment for such service. This further restricts the availability of some potentially excellent caregivers or relief help.

CHAPTER NINE

Letter to My Sons

My dear Derek, Jarret and Travis,

You have been so loved from the moment you were born and will be for all eternity. Derek, now that you have a son of your own, you know how intense that love can be. This love that you give is really a gift you give yourself.

Your father and I nourished you all physically, emotionally, intellectually and spiritually. We supported each of you in both large and small endeavors. We were there for you in both happy and sad times. We are very proud of who you have become. Your spirit of love, gentleness and courage are obvious to those who know you. You continue to shower us with pride in your accomplishments. This is the gift that I refer to that you give yourself. This is the legacy that your father and I leave to each of you.

You have had to face one of the biggest challenges of your life, that of losing a parent. This will prepare you to handle other challenges with ease. Christy lost her mother when she was only sixteen months old, and many others have lost parents at a tender age. We can be grateful for the time we have had together.

When I leave my physical body for my spiritual body, know that I will always be near in spirit. Life is but a blink in time and it won't be long before we will be re-united in the heavenly kingdom.

When we are young, we tend to focus more on the things of this earth and sometimes leave God on the back burner. I would like to encourage you to keep Him foremost in your mind and reflect Him in your spirit. God is our strength and through Him we can do all things. My hope and prayer is that you will each attain a level of spiritual maturity that will come from daily prayer and reflection on bible reading, living your faith and yes, going to church. You were created for a special mission in life and as you tune into the stillness of your soul and hear Gods voice, you will know what that mission is.

I have no doubt that you will each do well in life and be filled with true joy. I also know that if your dad should get sick, you will be there for him as he was for me. When your children see this, they will do the same for you. This is what love is all about.

Remember that success is not measured by how much you accumulate on earth. That is man's definition and it differs from God. True success is when you love God with your whole heart and soul and love others as He loves us. This will give you true joy and peace within. You have each expressed your belief on this subject and what I hear makes me happy. You each have good beliefs and values that will pass on to your children.

You know how much I love children and I would ask you to remind my present and future grandchildren how much they are loved by me. You also know how much I wanted a daughter and now I have Christy, who is like a daughter to me. I am so very proud of her and grateful that she came into our life. Please remind her that she holds a special place in my heart.

Our family has been blessed to have had such an enriched life with so many beautiful memories. Please continue the traditions and family dinners every Sunday for as often and as long as you can. These are special times to shut out the distractions of the world and bond as a family. You have many photo albums to remind you of our lives, growing together. Parenting was a learning experience for us just as it was a growing experience for you.

Derek and Christy, we are very proud of your parenting skills and instincts. Jarret and Travis, I know that you two have great paternal instincts and will also be wonderful fathers. Each of you is filled with so much love and all those whose lives you touch will be better for having known you.

Derek, you are 29 years old as I write this. You have been blessed with a beautiful wife, daughter and son. As a husband, you are very caring and considerate and share in the workload. As a father, you are playful and spend time with your children, which they will always remember. As a friend, you are genuine and a bit of a prankster. Your sense of humor and good disposition will keep the zest in all your relationships and keep the days bright. As a son, I could not be more proud of you.

You are very talented with your music and composing. I hope you will pursue it. You also are talented and creative with your hands. There are many opportunities awaiting you.

Jarret, you are now 26 years old. Your quiet, reserved nature is calming and noteworthy. What you have to say is always well thought out before you speak. Your gentle, caring and conscientious ways will serve you well in all your relationships as a friend, husband and father. Your loving and compassionate nature is evident whenever one is in your presence. Words cannot express how much your father and I have enjoyed your handmade cards throughout the years. As a student, you have excelled at the top and made us very proud. Your future looks bright and holds a lot of promise.

I am grateful for the trips we have been on, just you and me. We got to really know each other and appreciate our differences. You will have those beautiful memories to cherish.

Travis, you are 20 years old as I write this. You left home when you were 16 to pursue your hockey career. Next week you will be flying to visit Cornell University. You have had to deal with many challenges on your own, while living on the island. You are far beyond your years in maturity. You have excelled, not only in hockey, but also academically. Your brothers have accused you of asking too many questions, but there is nothing wrong with an inquisitive mind. You told me you learned to ask your mind the questions, which will give you the right answers. You have a great sense of humor and it is no wonder that you have so many friends, both near and far. Your magnetic personality will serve you well in all your relationships. You have a great deal of compassion and your warm loving nature flows from within. One can see your passion for living, which makes it a pleasure to be in your company. You are not only a leader on your team, but also a leader in your life. Your future looks very promising and many doors will be open to you. I know you will be all right on your own. Always know that wherever you are, I am with you in spirit. I am very proud of your accomplishments.

I have been thinking of a lasting gift for each of you. A gift that would keep on giving, which is a prayer I made up and say every day. It would be awesome to be united whenever we pray this prayer.

"Come Holy Spirit and dwell in my heart. Guide me in my relationship with you. Take away anything that would separate me from you. Oh God, you are my refuge and strength. Grant me the wisdom, courage and patience to deal with the challenges in my life. Guide me in my thoughts, words and deeds for this day, so they may glorify you. I thank you for the many blessings in my life. (then I name all the people who were in my life that day) I also thank you for the abundance of food, freedom and the beauty of nature that surrounds me. Amen

In your times of sadness and sorrow, think of our many treasured memories and know that I will always be near in spirit. I love you with all my heart.

Love,

Mom

CHAPTER TEN

Letters from Family & Friends

The following letters have been selected from many that I have received. I have chosen them to share with the readers of this book for the following reasons:

When one is afflicted with a fatal disease, it is difficult to comprehend how much pain and suffering one can bear, more than anyone can imagine.

When we choose to live our dying, we not only learn a lot about ourselves, but we also touch many people's lives, many that we have never even met.

I am so very grateful to the many that have written to me. It is a great shot in the arm.

The second reason is about showing our appreciation and love to all every day, because we do no know when our time has come. Why wait until after a person's death to proclaim what you admired and respected about that person? Why not tell people how you feel about them while they are alive and able to hear those things themselves? It is important to show love and appreciation throughout your whole life.

Lastly, I hope these letters will provide encouragement and inspiration to the afflicted.

A Letter to Evelyn from her Mother

Now that you've read Evelyn's book I want to share my thoughts and feelings with you.

I chose to go on this journey with Evelyn. God had a plan for me. And that's my mission to fulfill. My life has completely changed since I heard the devastating news about Evelyn's terminal disease, ALS. I left my home and moved in with her family. All these worldly things didn't matter anymore. I wanted to share the little time we still have together and that is more important now.

I will always love and cherish those memories. They are so very special to me. I am her mother – her caregiver and a life long friend. I went every step forward and downward with her. I see her so completely helpless and so dependent on us. It breaks my heart to watch her frail body and limbs hang so lifeless. I hear her cries of frustration, which come from her soul. She is so hopelessly trapped in her body. I want to be in there with her to comfort and share her pain. I turn to God and ask for help that I'll be able to endure the pain and suffering my daughter is going through. Everyday I see her getting weaker. My heart aches to watch my daughter die slowly before my eyes. I want to hang on to her as long as I can. On the other hand, I don't want her to suffer so long. I don't understand God's plan. I think he is testing us to see how strong our faith is.

Evelyn is full of courage and love. I know God is with her, to give her strength to handle the difficult times. I go to bed at night tired, drained and stressed. My heart is heavy, my mind darts in all directions. I hear her moan at night waiting to be turned. So I bravely turn to God and ask for a peaceful night's rest for all of us. Tears flow in silence and I pray so this nightmare would end. But in the morning it's a reality. So we start another day with God's help. I see Evelyn with sparkling eyes and a smile. Then I forget my aches and I begin the day with continually wiping her mouth, nose, and eyes and watch her hands, head and itchy places. I smile, give her a loving hug or touch and we go on.

Evelyn is my first born. Indeed a gift from God. She was so precious and beautiful to us. She brought us so much love and laughter. She was a perfectionist and an inspiration to all around her. She was so warm and made everyone feel so welcome in her home. I love her deeply and I'm so very proud of her. I admire her inner strength and courage and will never forget her lovely smile.

She is so lucky to have such a compassionate and caring husband and three loving sons, as well as so many friends and family who care. She gets so much help and so many cards, gifts and phone calls, so many visits. I feel God is around us helping every step of the way. I know her mind is filled with love and prayer. The frustration must be so unbearable because I feel it by watching her. She is so weak and frail now, she needs a lot of help to finish her book of awareness.

We place our trust in God. There is no hope, no help to get better. I want to reach out to help and I cannot. I know where Evelyn is going is a better place and she'll walk again, and do everything she wants to and no more suffering or pain. When I go to another household, I feel sunshine, warmth, laughter and happiness and the world goes on as if nothing matters. But it's different when I come home. It feels dull, cool, quiet. Pain around you, but very spiritual and close to God.

I thank God every day that I'm healthy, and that I am able to help wherever I can. And I do it all for the honor and glory of God.

Dec. 8/98

Dearest Evelyn,

Words cannot express the sincere feelings I have for you at this special time. I wish I could wrap my arms around you and change everything, but God has a plan for each one of us, as I'm sure He has a special plan for you. You have been such an inspiration for me with your incredible courage and undying faith. This also shows through in your boys. Evelyn, you and Larry have a beautiful family. There is a lot to be learned from all of you.

I wish to tell you once again how much I admire you and truly cherish your friendship. You have always been a wonderful friend and I am a better person for having known you. You and Larry are our family's most treasured friends. Keep up the good fight Evelyn. Until we meet again. Have a blessed Christmas.

Love,

Adeline

Dear Evelyn,

I was studying for my French exam this evening when I noticed your newspaper article in my dad's office. I couldn't carry on with my French without thinking of you and your incredible battle. I know my whole family admires your courage and bravery, but I think your attitude is the thing that stands out. You are choosing to live your life by looking at the cup half-full and choosing to be better rather than bitter. Larry, I also admire your continuation as a caring loving husband through these tough times. We pray for you a lot and I believe that God is with you every step of the way. I turned sixteen in January and just got my driver's license (look out!). We will be heading through Calgary on the way back from Saskatoon. I hope to have a nice visit with both of you, and hopefully your boys if they're coming home. Hope to see you soon and we send our love.

Sincerely,
Josh Heinrichs

This letter was written by Kelly Eaton, whose mother Betty Norman died of ALS in July 1997

October 14, 1998
Dear Evelyn,

You and Larry are in my thoughts so often and I just wanted to send some warm thoughts your way.

I saw you on the news the other night and was very impressed and proud of what you are personally doing for ALS awareness. Many people in my community saw that broadcast and mentioned it to me. I proudly said that you were one of our special run ambassadors last year. You and Larry did an excellent job of demonstrating the struggles of the disease – but in a "positive" way. I was very encouraged to see your smiling face and listen to the progress on the book you're writing. Mom's progress was so rapid and extreme – we rarely had any opportunities together to do anything but deal with her disease. I'm so thankful she was able to at least experience the excitement around the Run.

I'm excited about the book you are writing and send my encouragement to you. It's another thing that I felt I missed out on – what was going through Mom's mind through all this. I think your story will be a huge contribution to the awareness and understanding of ALS. I know you have lots of supporters, but I too will help in whatever it takes to get it published and printed! So don't fret about those details.

I spoke with Larry this morning about how you are doing. It is such a difficult path you are travelling on —my heart really aches for you. Keep up that incredible positive attitude you have and rely on your faith in God to give you strength. The best and most simple advice I ever was given was to "take one day at a time". It seems silly but it was the only way I got through the year of Mom's illness.

Heroes in this world take on many forms and functions. Like my Mom, you are exhibiting the courage, strength and selflessness of a true hero that will be remembered always! I pray for its continuance and for peace for you.

With warmest wishes,

Kelly

Dec. 1/98

Dear Evelyn,

I wish so often we could have a good conversation like we used to. It seems so utterly unbelievable that in just two and a half years, this disease has completely debilitated your body. But not your fighting spirit, your dignity, nor your faith and love of others.

Besides learning how devastating ALS is, I have learned so much more from you through your courageous efforts in dealing with the constant losses of mobility, speech and independence. All of us, especially the kids have learned a lot from you regarding the value of a loving and supportive family, the relative unimportance of material things and the absolute necessity for faith in God. Also you have taught us to appreciate everyday, to talk less and listen more. I wake up some mornings and feel guilty for taking so much for granted. I think, now

I can get up and dress myself, brush my hair, eat breakfast and drive to work. I can write a letter, talk on the phone and hug my family. I can do all these things myself everyday and you can not. I wonder how you find the strength to keep going against such adversity. I wonder how you must hurt inside, if you feel angry, if you yearn to talk. You may not have a voice, but your eyes reach my heart and soul.

Larry and Mom are doing such an outstanding job as your primary caregivers. Having watched what is required for your daily care, I believe that no institutional caregivers could ever provide what they're doing. Why does our health care system not provide more adequately for such demanding and intensive level of care in the home when it is so needed? And your other caregivers are remarkable too! They give so much of themselves and seem to have grown personally and professionally from their intense experience with you and ALS.

I admire you for your determination in writing a book despite the very difficult and wearisome process of dictating the pages letter by letter using a spellboard and scribers. You really leave a memorable legacy especially for your sons, who already have shown such courage, responsibility and love.

I feel very fortunate to be around you. You exemplify the love, hope and faith in God that we all strive for in life. Your earthly sacrifice has surely earned you a place in heaven and I believe our Dad is proudly waiting with open arms.

With much love and admiration,
Your sister, Vel

August, 1998
Dear Evelyn

Knowing I was coming to see you today, I felt compelled to put some thoughts on paper.

It's hard for me to believe that we first met twenty-four years ago, when Derek and Jeff were in kindergarten together. A wonderful friendship grew from there, including a business relationship. In the past week I've thought a lot about that relationship and how it affected my life.

As you know, my marital situation was in turmoil, but I was afraid of leaving the security the boys and I had. Then I met you. You introduced me to Nutri-Metics and my whole world changed. I knew then that I could support my boys and myself and was then able to start a new and wonderful life for all of us. You were indeed a catalyst and I believe your presence in my life at that time was no accident. God works in mysterious ways.

In the many months we spent together, I watched you fulfill your many roles with great admiration and respect. I envied your lack of "baggage" and the relationship you had with your parents and siblings. But what I most recall is how, by observing you, I learned to "go the extra mile".

When I entertain, and people rave about how they love to come to my home because it's always such a treat, I know that I learned that from you and I have reflected on that many times over the last several years. You were the perfect hostess!

It's hard to comprehend why a woman as beautiful and vibrant as you is having to endure such a horrifying disease. There are no answers to that question. I'm sure that if love and prayers would heal your body, you'd be well in a heartbeat.

I am grateful that I can share some time with you and be given the opportunity to let you know how profoundly you touched me so many years ago.

May God give you and your family the strength you all need through this most difficult time.

You are in my thoughts and prayers.

Much love,

Judy

January 5, 1999

Dear Evelyn,

For me, this letter is long overdue. Yesterday after reading the article about your book, I knew I could procrastinate no longer. You have been on my mind almost daily since I heard of your illness, and every Sunday I say a prayer for you and your family at church.

You truly are an amazing woman and after reading the article in The Herald about you writing a book, I didn't want to miss the opportunity to tell you.

When I first joined Nutri-Metics, I believe it was a Godsend that you were my sponsor. I know I didn't stay with it long, but as you know, our paths were to meet again. When I rejoined Nutri-Metics, as a consultant for the second time, I now look back and know I had an alternative motive. That was to be near you!

What do I mean by that? Well Evelyn, I wanted to be near a person like yourself who was so positive and who had everything anyone would want – success and a wonderful family. You see Evelyn, at the time I rejoined Nutri-Metics I was going through an extremely difficult time in my life, personally as well as with my marriage.

Going to the weekly meetings and listening to you speak and just being near you to absorb your energy and love of life was exactly what I needed to help me get over that "life hurdle". I knew you wanted more from me from the business aspect, for that I do apologize. I do want you to know that the encouragement I received from you was a far better gift and now I read about the challenges you face in life, and you still continue to give to others, in the form of a book.

You truly are a remarkable woman and **I will always be thankful to have had you in my life**. You are an inspiration to those who do not even have any challenges that compare to yours, but still feel life is treating them unfairly. Sometimes when I think about it, I can't even express how I feel, I am so overwhelmed.

For some unknown reason, God chooses a journey for us for which we may not be prepared. I believe He has chosen you for your journey because He knew how strong you were and that you would help to bring awareness to this disease (ALS).

I also want to admit that I am taking the coward's way out by writing this letter as I don't think I have the courage to see you personally. The last thing you need is some emotional, weeping person on your doorstep.

Evelyn, thank you for all that you have given me and as I said before, I am so thankful that I had the opportunity to have you as part of my life. You will always be an inspiration to me.

My thoughts, love and prayers are with you and your family.

Carol Bjornsen

The following are letters written to Larry and Evelyn on their 31st wedding anniversary, November 11, 1998 by their son, Jarret.

My Sweet Mom,

What words can I possibly put down on paper to express how much I look up to you, how much I am inspired by your courage, mental and physical will and unending faith. And how much I **love** you.

It is your strength I look to for guidance and clarity to understand what is real to me. . . and that is you – your love shared with Dad. . . and that showered upon your boys, the sons whom you have so unselfishly raised (especially that middle son who you've spoiled on all those Nutri-Metics trips!) Mom, I cherish those excursions we've had together, getting to know each other, becoming best friends and I enjoy our excursions together now - looking into each other's eyes. . . able to somehow understand one another 'non-verbally' with that uniting 'blink" of the eye we so often give each other.

Mom, you have always offered your arms for my support, your ears for my concerns and your heart for my tears. And now you continue to give – sharing your unending strength with me and all who surround you. I carry your lessons of love, courage and faith close to my heart, hoping I will one day learn how to reflect them as you do!

So now we must embrace each new day, be patient with its offerings and use our 'love for one-another' and our faith – to guide us through the challenges presented.

I love you Mom. Happy Anniversary.

Love,

Jarret

My father,

It is hard for me to truly describe my 'aweness' at your continued acts of. . . devotion, self-sacrifice and the gentleness within your heart. Dad, you radiate so much love and kindness to your family. It seems you have always been the "ultimate CAREGIVER". You seem to make sure everyone is provided for – before tending to your own needs, and often maybe not at all.

I look at you and can often see your pain and frustration in providing endless care to your wife, partner, best friend of 31 years – my sweet mother.

Derek described it best by saying "you are my hero" because you are, dad. I look up to you with so much admiration and respect. I hope I will someday be able to provide for my family in the ways you have modeled.

Dad, please continue to find the patience in these times of struggle. I am here for you and mom in any way I can possibly help (and I know I could do so much more).

Dad, don't forget to take TIME – for you – only you – so you don't ever lose that crazy sense of humor or that gentle spirit that holds this family together.

I love you Dad.

Jarret